Wives and Midwives

Comparative Studies of Health Systems and Medical Care

General Editor
CHARLES LESLIE

John M. Janzen, *The Quest for Therapy in Lower Zaire*

Paul U. Unschuld, *Medical Ethics in Imperial China: A Study in Historical Anthropology*

Margaret M. Lock, *East Asian Medicine in Urban Japan: Varieties of Medical Experience*

Jeanie Schmit Kayser-Jones, *Old, Alone, and Neglected: Care of the Aged in Scotland and in the United States*

Arthur Kleinman, *Patients and Healers in the Context of Culture: An Exploration of the Borderland Between Anthropology, Medicine and Psychiatry*

Stephen J. Kunitz, *Disease Change and the Role of Medicine: The Navajo Experience*

Carol Laderman, *Wives and Midwives: Childbirth and Nutrition in Rural Malaysia*

Wives and Midwives

Childbirth and Nutrition in Rural Malaysia

Carol Laderman

University of California Press

Berkeley · Los Angeles · London

University of California Press
Berkeley and Los Angeles, California
University of California Press, Ltd.
London, England
Copyright © 1983 by The Regents of the University of California
Library of Congress Cataloging in Publication Data

Library of Congress Cataloging in Publication Data

Laderman, Carol.
Wives and midwives.

(Comparative studies of health systems and medical care)
Bibliography: p. 247
Includes index.
1. Malays (Asian people)—Medicine.
2. Birth customs—Malaysia—Terengganu.
3. Food habits—Malaysia—Terengganu.
4. Puerperium—Nutritional aspects.
5. Kampong Merchang (Terengganu)—Social life and customs.
1. Title.   II. Series.   [DNLM: 1. Midwifery.
2. Pregnancy.   3. Nutrition surveys—Malaysia.
4. Rural health—Malaysia.
5. Anthropology, Cultural—Malaysia. GN635.M4 L154c]
GN635.M4L33   1983   306'.46   83-47664
ISBN 0-520-04924-1

Printed in the United States of America
1 2 3 4 5 6 7 8 9

For Gabriel, my husband and best friend.

Contents

Contents

[viii]

Contents

Acknowledgments

My thanks are owing, most of all, to the people of Merchang, who taught my son in their excellent village school and educated his mother in the daily exchanges of social life. They generously reassured me that "Carol isn't really stupid, she's just ignorant," and did their best to improve my understanding. From the first day, our neighbors welcomed us with friendship and patience. They allowed us to share their lives, celebrating with them at births and marriages and mourning with them at sickness and death. The Malays have a proverb: "Debts of gold can be repaid, debts of kindness are carried to the grave." I can never properly repay the kindness of Sapiah, who taught me the duties and rewards of midwifery, of Tok Daud, who explained the mysteries of the healing art, of Pak Long Awang, my Malay foster father, of Noh, my landlady, cook and friend, and of all the women who let me weigh their food and take their blood.

I would like to acknowledge my debt to the government of Malaysia for allowing me to pursue my research in their beautiful country. Thanks are due especially to the Institute for Medical Research and its director, Dr. George DeWitt, to Dr. Y. H. Chong of the Division of Nutrition, to Dr. Albert Rudnick of the International Center for Medical Research, and to the Division of

Rural Health. Encik Zahid bin Muda, the District Officer of Marang District, was unfailingly helpful and courteous, as were the *penghulu* and *ketua kampung* of Merchang. Dr. Kuljit Singh, the director of the General Hospital in Kuala Trengganu, was instrumental in helping me find a research site, and authorized his staff to teach me the technique of blood collection. The hospital's Department of Pathology, under the direction of Dr. Manjit Singh, performed some of the blood chemistry tests.

Maudene Nelson, of the Institute of Human Nutrition at Columbia University, with remarkable generosity, contributed many hours of painstaking, tedious work, analyzing the nutritional content of the diets I collected. S. Pathansali, director of the Fisheries Research Institute in Penang, assisted me in the identification of local fish, and Prof. Bernard Gordon of Northeastern University, and Drs. C. Lamont Smith and James Atz of the American Museum of Natural History, helped me identify the fish implicated in toxic reactions. Prof. Benjamin C. Stone, of the Department of Botany, University of Malaya, identified the wild vegetables and fruits of Merchang.

I thank the Danforth Foundation, which supported me through all my years at graduate school, and the following institutions that supported my research: The Social Science Research Council, The National Institute of Mental Health (Training Grant 5 F31 MHO532-03), and the University of California International Center for Medical Research, through research grant A1 10051 to the Department of Epidemiology and International Health, University of California, San Francisco, from the National Institute of Allergy and Infectious Diseases, National Institutes of Health. I also thank Columbia University for their offer of a Traveling Fellowship.

My years at Columbia were happy and productive, largely due to the intelligence and humanity of my advisor, Prof. Alexander Alland, Jr. He believed in my ability to unravel the complexities of the humoral system, and did not hesitate to say so in print, long

Acknowledgments

before I, myself, was convinced. Profs. Conrad M. Arensberg and Clive Kessler generously shared their time and knowledge throughout my graduate career, as did Prof. Barbara Kirshenblatt-Gimblett, a good friend and incisive critic. My gratitude goes, as well to Prof. Rena Gropper of Hunter College, who first introduced me to anthropology. Her inspired teaching changed the course of my life. My debts to her and to all of my teachers are the kind that are "carried to the grave," but I hope that this book can, in some small measure, repay them.

I appreciate the many times my lifelong friend, Barbara Ribakove, read and commented on the various versions of this manuscript, and the invaluable criticism of my editor, Prof. Charles Leslie.

Finally, I would like to thank my family: my husband, Gabriel, and my sons, Raphael and Michael. They encouraged me through many years of study, both undergraduate and graduate, although this demanded many adjustments and sacrifices on their part. They accompanied me to a foreign land, learned a new language, and adapted themselves to another culture. They never stopped believing in the value of my research, or in my capacity to reduce our shared experience to words. To all those who helped me, I say *"terima kasih,"* the Malay thank you that literally means "accept love," and to my family I say *"kasih sayang,"* all my love to you.

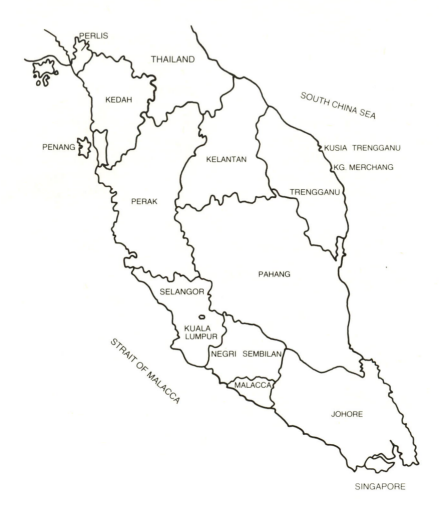

PENINSULAR MALAYSIA

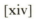

· 1 ·

Introduction to the Problem
and the People

The strength of anthropology lies within a paradox. The broad philosophical and theoretical concerns of anthropology must be approached through studies of a particular people, living in a particular time and place. But in order to understand the particular, we must approach it from a generalist viewpoint. The specific nature of our inquiries cannot be allowed to limit our field of investigation. Data must be collected even in those areas which at first glance seem to impinge only peripherally upon the problem. For example, understanding a people's dietary habits requires a knowledge of their economy and ecology, as well as their religious, social, and aesthetic ideologies. An analysis of childbirth practices must include an investigation into sex roles, rules of marriage and divorce, and the status and training of childbirth attendants, as well as the medical system of which these practices are a part.

Cultural adaptation—the ways in which cultural traits influence the successful interaction between a population and its environment—has been a long-term concern of anthropologists. I have approached this problem through ever-narrowing specifics: first, traditional Malay medicine; further, pregnancy and

[1]

childbirth among rural Malays on the east coast of peninsular Malaysia; and finally, dietary beliefs and practices associated with childbirth in a parish of Trengganu. Thus, although the underlying question is "How adaptive are traditional cultures?" the problem this study confronts is "How adaptive is the traditional postpartum diet among a population of rural Malays in a particular parish of the state of Trengganu?" Thus phrased, the question should be of primary interest only to those concerned with the specifics of contemporary Malay health. Before I could arrive at an assessment of this seemingly narrow problem I had to consider questions of great import for cross-cultural studies.

One such question is the relationship between belief and behavior. We are all aware of discrepancies between the real and the ideal, between what people say they should do, what they claim to have done, and what they are observed doing. A major trend in contemporary anthropology is an inquiry into the ways in which people manipulate their ideologies to achieve valued ends. Earlier accounts assumed that people in tribal societies automatically gave political allegiance to an individual or group according to their expressed ideology. This notion was challenged by Barth (1959), who showed that among a particular tribal people, the Swat Pathans, the authority system is maintained through a series of individual choices. His findings were widened by later investigators (notably Bailey 1969) into an investigation of the means by which competitors for scarce prizes, economic as well as political, deviate from normative rules in all societies. Religious ideology is no longer expected to be automatically translated into behavior. In a study of Thai peasants, for example, Phillips found that fewer men fulfilled their religious obligation of monastic ordination than chose to ignore it (1965, 1969). Kinship, too, has ceased to be seen as a monolithic structure. Regardless of the formal kinship system, people activate and deactivate kinship links, claiming distant relations as kin if they are important enough to warrant such inclusion, and denying relationships to those they would like to distance (Schneider 1968; see also Lindenbaum 1979; Siskind 1973). The climate of opinion in much of present-day anthropology is that, rather than being merely actors who play out their roles according to a prepared cultural script, people innovate, interpret, cheat and rationalize their behavior.

The concept of behavioral flexibility in the face of ideology, however, is not current in many discussions of food behavior. Although people have been recognized as practical and even clever in their social and cultural manipulations of other areas of their lives, they are often represented as rigidly following traditional dietary rules which may drastically limit the utilization of otherwise available foods, even though this may lead to malnutrition (e.g., Foster and Anderson 1978:271–276; Cassidy 1980, 1981; Wilson 1970, 1973; Wolff 1965). The flexibility with which Malays interpret their food ideology, as reported in this book, brings into question those studies which posit a simple equation between ideology and dietary behavior. The correspondence is infinitely more complex, involving the invocation of "rules to break rules" which assure the continued integrity of the symbolic system by patterning what might otherwise seem like rifts in its fabric. Beyond this, since incorporation of variation into the behavioral model can maximize a population's adaptive potential in the event of social or environmental change (see Alland 1970:3–4), the study of the amount and quality of such variation in regard to nutrition can be a powerful tool for the assessment of biocultural adaptation.

An investigation of food ideology and behavior can provide material for a discussion of the nature of symbolic systems and their relation to empirical reality. Scholars have long speculated about the meanings and functions of food taboos. In recent times two schools of thought have been prominent in their analysis. They have been explained by symbolists as systems created for the avoidance of ambiguity or cognitive dissonance (e.g., Douglas 1966) or as vehicles for embodying social ideas metaphorically

[3]

(e.g., Tambiah 1969), and by materialists as lessons learned from the environment (e.g., Harris 1966:1977). These approaches reflect two conflicting paradigms of anthropological theory which Sahlins (1976) characterizes as culture and practical reason. The former is based on the idea that human action is mediated by cultural design, while the latter conceives of the cultural order as a codification of pragmatic action. This has been viewed as an unbridgeable opposition, yet an analysis of food restrictions can demonstrate how the rationale underlying their formulations may simultaneously give symbolic coherence to the values and world view of the culture and provide signposts for behavior.[1] Although symbolic systems are never merely reflections of the natural world, within them we may discover biological and eco-logical codes, and models which can simplify the decision-making process (see Lindenbaum 1977; Gladwin 1979). Such is the case in two Malay conceptual systems (discussed in detail in chap. 3) which pattern the diet, particularly during sickness and in the postpartum period. In each, the symbolic logic of the system is reinforced at strategic points by empirical perceptions. Demon-strating the interrelationship of symbolic and empirical logic in this particular instance should encourage an integrated approach not only to the analysis of food avoidances, but to larger issues concerning the nature of cultural patterning and human thought.

Medical anthropology has a great potential for combining within a subdiscipline the four-field approach of American an-thropology, which calls upon studies of physical anthropology, ethnography, linguistics and archeology to present a picture of the human condition in the round. Its potential is denied if it is allowed to break off from the mainstream and develop its own idiosyncrasies and special concerns. Medical anthropology can be used not only as a gateway into the study of biocultural adaptation (Alland 1966), but as a means of understanding the workings of culture in ways not dissimilar to those of other subdisciplines, such as political or economic anthropology. The association of

[4]

anthropology with medicine, however, in a society which encourages a conceptual split between "hard science" and "humanism," has resulted in a dichotomized rather than an integrated subfield of a discipline that prides itself on holism. Studies have stressed either ethnomedicine, concentrating on the form and meaning given to medical problems by members of the studied community, or biomedicine, applying the knowledge and viewpoint of Western biological science and medicine to specify the level and distribution of disease within the community. Each of these approaches, separately, is incomplete. The ethnomedical approach has been characterized by impressionistic data regarding health, and the biomedical approach, while providing hard data, lacks the cultural base in which this data must be imbedded to be truly meaningful. Good methodology must combine objective measures with a knowledge of cultural categories and local terminology. Lacking such understanding, it is impossible to formulate the questions which will produce the data which an investigator is seeking.

Arthur Kleinman's study of medicine in Taiwan (1980) is outstanding for his systematic attempt to follow patients treated by indigenous healers, not only to determine the theory and practice of traditional medicine, but also to assess its effectiveness. Almost three-quarters of all sickness episodes recorded in his survey, however, were not treated by medical practitioners, but were handled by the patient himself or in consultation with his family (1980:310). Although this sphere of health care, which Kleinman calls the popular sector, is the largest part of any system, it is the least studied and most poorly understood (1980:50). Discussing the difficulty of describing these transactions, much less determining their value, Kleinman states, "There is no precise time when they occur, nor do they end with the finality of a healing ritual or a modern clinical consultation" (1980:310).

As a general statement, this is undoubtedly true, yet there is an area of traditional health care primarily in the popular sector which has a clearly delineated beginning and end, whose rules can be clearly stated and whose duration is short enough to allow an investigator to monitor patients' actual behavior as well as eliciting normative statements. In rural Malaysia, childbirth, the event that initiates this health behavior, is supervised by a professional medical practitioner, a midwife who, in her role as ritual practitioner, also releases her patient from the observances specific to the puerperium. Within the postpartum period, however, primary care rests normally with the patient and her family. Since this period is so neatly demarcated, it is possible to determine by objective means the health consequences of following traditional dietary rules, provided that a base line has been obtained early in each pregnancy.

An anthropologist, working alone, might be able to encompass many of the variables which feed into an understanding of this problem. Yet, no matter how satisfying an ethnomedical study may be, it is incomplete unless there are objective standards for discussing the effects of these variables upon the diet, upon the outcome of childbirth, and upon people's health. An undertaking of this nature presupposes collaboration with other disciplines, especially when the anthropologist, like myself, has had no previous medical training (although before the project was over I had learned to draw blood, massage a patient, analyze a diet, and deliver a baby). Its success depends upon contributions from a multiplicity of sources: nutritionists, blood pathologists, medical personnel both traditional and hospital-based, ichthyologists, an oceanographer, and a botanist.

Data derived from blood serum nutrient and dietary analyses provide measures of adaptation on the individual level, and indications of the effectiveness of health care in the popular sector of this population. These objective measures, combined with pertinent ethnographic data derived from participant observation, extensive interviewing, and historical and ecological studies, present an articulated picture of a portion of a traditional medical system as it operates simultaneously on a cultural and physiological level.

Since the focus of the study was on the postpartum diet, it was important to know what the normal diet was like in all its seasonal permutations, and whether the diet during pregnancy varied from the nonpregnant diet, to be able to appreciate the changes taking place during the puerperium. Bare facts about the diet could not be understood outside of their ecological, economic and symbolic framework. The postpartum period, itself, could not be discussed without an understanding of the traditional medical system, the social, ritual, and biological functions of pregnancy and childbirth within this cultural context, and the roles and statuses of patients and practitioners. The exigencies of the study dictate the structure of this book. After painting a picture in broad strokes of the people and the area in which this research took place, I will discuss the two major protagonists of this work: the women of Merchang and its ecology. The subjects of this book, childbirth and nutrition, bring together the reproductive aspects of both human beings and the land on which they live. I will examine the influences of the environment on nutrition, and of the symbolic system on behavior. After presenting a picture in depth of the world view which infuses the lives of these rural Malays with meaning, I will discuss the effects upon maternal health of this nexus of ecology and belief.

MERCHANG, THE PLACE AND ITS PEOPLE

Since I wanted to compare the indigenous medical system with cosmopolitan medicine as it is practiced in Malaysia, I sought a research site in which traditional healers and midwives were active, and access to cosmopolitan medicine was possible. I chose the state of Trengganu, where geographic location and a deliberate policy of political isolation have caused it to remain the most traditionally Malay of the eleven states of peninsular Malaysia.

Although Great Britain had been a power on the Malay Peninsula since 1786, it was not until 1910 that Trengganu abandoned its isolationist stance and signed an agreement allowing a British officer to reside in the state capital, thereby becoming an Unfederated Malay State (Sheppard 1949). Geographically, Trengganu remained relatively isolated until the middle of this century. Its sixteen rivers, flowing into the South China Sea, had to be crossed by ferry. At high tide and during the monsoon the ferries lay idle, and heavy rains (over 140" annually), flooding the highway that connects the east and west coasts, effectively cut Trengganu off from contact with the rest of the country for several months each year. It was not until the mid-1960s that the ferries were replaced by bridges and portions of the highway rebuilt further inland to lessen flooding.

Unlike many of the west coast states, Trengganu had no heavy influx of Chinese and Indian workers, imported by the British to work in tin mines and rubber plantations. The proportion of Malays in the populations of such western states as Penang and Selangor hovers around 30 percent while that of Trengganu is close to 94 percent (Population and Housing Census of Malaysia 1970). This preponderance of ethnic Malays, and Trengganu's long history of political and geographic isolation, are reflected in the dialect spoken and the customs observed. Trengganu dialect includes fewer foreign words than any other spoken on the peninsula (Brown 1935:1–2), and has retained in its everyday vocabulary words which have become archaic or have disappeared from other Malay dialects (Brown 1970:xiv). Customs and practices which once were widespread throughout the peninsula, but which have vanished or been strongly modified in other states, have endured in Trengganu.

The parish (*mukim*) I chose as my research site is equidistant from two urban centers. It is possible to reach the hospital in Kuala Dungun or Kuala Trengganu (each a distance of 25 miles), and the Health Center in Marang (13 miles away), by boarding a

[8]

bus which passes by several times a day, or by hiring the parish's one taxi. There has been a government midwife in attendance in the parish since 1958 and a midwife's clinic since 1962. However, this is an area in which traditional midwives (*bidan kampung*) and indigenous medical practitioners (*bomoh*) carry on a thriving practice. My choice was particularly felicitous since, with the luck that seems to accrue to most anthropologists, I rented a house belonging to the son of a *bidan kampung*; the bidan herself lived directly across the road.

Merchang (the name is used both for the parish and its central village) is located on the coast of the South China Sea, five degrees north of the equator.[2] Unlike many other coastal village-hamlet complexes, including those in the vicinity, Merchang has not only been settled close to the major highway which runs parallel to the coastline, but extends approximately three miles inland to meet the jungle, which is gradually being cleared by loggers and for agriculture. Secondary and tertiary dirt roads leading away from the highway culminate in a mud and stick path erected over a swamp which, except during the monsoon when it is completely under water, connects the jungle-outpost kampung with the rest of the world.

Each of the mukim's hamlets has its own coffeehouse-cum-shop, just as each has its own *surau* (house of prayer), but for major purchases and communal prayer on Friday, the Islamic sabbath, people come to Merchang's center where the general stores, public meeting house and mosque are to be found.

With the exception of a handful of Chinese storekeepers and sawmill operators, all the villagers are Malay and therefore Muslim. According to the Malaysian constitution, a Malay is one who professes the Muslim religion, habitually speaks the Malay language, and conforms to Malay customs (Hamid 1964:180). Trengganu is known as *Dar al-Iman*, the Land of Believers, and its people are celebrated for their piety. But alongside Islamic orthodoxy are beliefs in semidivine characters from the Hindu-

[9]

derived shadow play and a variety of spirits, all of whom figure prominently in Malay theories of disease causation.

Due to its inland extension, Merchang's ecology includes seashore, river, swamp, primary and secondary forest, and cultivated land with both sandy and rich soil. Its coastal location and the availability of land make fishing, agriculture, and logging the major occupations. The climate is tropical, with mean temperatures hovering around 85 degrees in the day, except during the monsoon when temperatures can drop to the sixties.

In general, the farther the kampung is from the highway, the more dispersed its settlement. Some families in the jungle outpost kampung live a quarter of a mile from their nearest neighbors. Houses, occasionally woven of pandanus leaves but usually made of wood planks, are built on stilts two to seven feet from the ground, preventing flooding during the monsoon, permitting the circulation of air during hot weather, and providing space for storage of tools and coconuts. Children play under houses, especially during bad weather, and chickens run back and forth, clucking under the floorboards. The height of the entrance discourages snakes and monitor lizards from invading the house but affords no protection from frequent intrusions of cats and chickens, and an occasional visit from a goat.

The floorboards are not flush. Space is deliberately left between them, not only for ventilation, but for the disposal of sweepings and other debris. Any food dropped on the floor goes down to feed the ever-vigilant chickens. Accidents of children who have not yet mastered toilet training are easy to clean with a bucket of water and a coconut husk. The ease of cleaning takes on considerable importance during childbirth, when the effluvia of delivery must be removed and the new mother and baby bathed inside the house.

Except in the case of newlyweds, it is rare to find a household lacking children. Malays consider such a home unbearably lonely. Grandparents and childless couples are often given children to raise by relatives with an abundance at home. The high incidence of divorce and remarriage makes it commonplace for children of more than one marriage to live with the current conjugal pair. Although most young couples start a new home of their own, they often build it near their parents' house. Neighbors do not, and are not expected to, offer much help beyond polite inquiry and moral support during illness, childbirth or other family crises, but close female relatives often nurse their kin or assist with young children and housework in an emergency. Wives and mothers must fit these services into a busy schedule.

WOMEN'S OCCUPATIONS

Women's work begins early and ends late. By 6 A.M. the ring of stone mortar against pestle resounds from most houses as the women prepare breakfast. The woodburning stove must be lit, the babies fed and bathed, and children supervised as they prepare for school. After the children have left, the housewife cleans the dishes with soap and cold well water, using sand to scour the pots and pans. Every day she must draw water from the well, pulling the bucket up hand over hand, for bathing, cooking, drinking, washing dishes, and laundry. Drinking water, in most families, is boiled and stored in bottles. Laundry must be washed, hung out to dry, and folded every day. The floors are swept daily and occasionally scrubbed on hands and knees with soap and water and a stiff brush. Garbage is burned every day and the area around the house is raked clean. Fish must be cleaned and gutted in preparation for the day's cooking. Although Malays eat three meals a day, the housewife usually cooks twice since the same meal is often served for both lunch and supper. Husbands returning from migratory labor are fussed over by their wives, who add to their chores by preparing favorite snacks (cf. Siegel 1969).

Frequently the housewife ends her day folding laundry after the children have gone to sleep. If her baby awakes during the

[11]

night, she puts it to the breast. Babies are usually nursed from one to as many as four years, if there are no younger siblings. A fractious baby is its mother's responsibility, and losing sleep over it does not excuse her from the next day's work. Women must be sick indeed before they abdicate their daily tasks.

Besides performing their household duties, most women spend part of the day cultivating the fields and/or tapping rubber. Their wages are lower than men's: a day's agricultural work pays a man M$5.00, a woman receives M$3.50. Fishing and lumbering, two of the more lucrative occupations, are closed to women. Male sawmill workers earn M$150 to 400 a month, while women's agricultural work rarely brings in more than M$70.00.

Even women with very young children work part of the day away from home, if they have a reliable babysitter, often a daughter whose household duties begin at an early age. From about the age of seven, girls are expected to help with cooking, laundry and child care. Their contribution to the household economy is so valuable that many girls are kept at home after finishing six years of elementary school rather than being allowed to join their brothers in junior high. They soon find another arena in which to practice the skills they learned at home. One-third marry within three years of leaving elementary school (see table 1), and three-fourths have been wed by the age of sixteen. Pregnancy soon follows (see table 2). By the time a woman is thirty-five she usually has five or more children (see table 3). Girls and boys are valued equally. No matter how many children a couple may have, if they are all the same sex the family is considered incomplete and a child of the unrepresented sex may be adopted.

MARRIAGE AND DIVORCE

For the majority of women and a large proportion of men, the first marriage will last throughout the spouses' lifetimes, but more

TABLE 1
AGE AT FIRST MARRIAGE

Women			Men		
12 years old	8%	(11)			
13	7	(9)			
14	17	(23)			
15	24	(36)	15 years old	4%	(4)
16	19	(26)	16	7	(7)
17	9	(13)	17	14	(15)
18	12	(17)	18	20	(21)
19	2	(2)	19	6	(6)
20	2	(2)	20	26	(27)
21	1	(1)	21	8	(8)
22	1	(1)	22	1	(1)
			23	1	(1)
			24	3	(3)
			25	11	(12)
	N = 141			N = 105	

than a third of the women and almost two-thirds of the men are serial monogamists (see table 4). This seeming discrepancy is owing to the fact that marriage partners are found without as well as within the immediate community. The record for serial marriage in Merchang went to a man with sixteen wives to his credit.

Most first marriages are still arranged by the parents of the bride and groom. Malays belong to the Shafi school of the orthodox, or Sunni, sect of Islam, a school that has been characterized as "definitely less favorable to women than the Hanafi or the Maliki" (Vesey-Fitzgerald 1931:16). Unlike a Hanafi girl, who may give herself in marriage after attaining puberty, a Shafi woman must have a guardian (*wali*) to give her away with her consent, if she is not a virgin, or without her consent, and even against her wishes, if she is a virgin. Girls are rarely compelled to marry, but I have heard of some who deliberately lost their

[13]

TABLE 2
AGE OF WOMEN AT FIRST PREGNANCY

12 years old	3%	(3)
13	2	(2)
14	12	(14)
15	18	(20)
16	20	(23)
17	14	(16)
18	14	(16)
19	7	(8)
20	7	(8)
21	0	
22	2	(2)
23	0	
24	1	(1)
25	1	(1)

N = 114

TABLE 3
NUMBER OF CHILDREN BY AGE OF MOTHER

	Less than 25	25–34	35–44	45 and over
1	46%	2.5%	0%	0%
2	33	2.5	3.5	11.5
3	8	14	15	18
4	8	22	11	6
5	4	22	22	18
6		20	11	11.5
7		14	18.5	11.5
8		2.5	7.5	11.5
9			7.5	11.5
10				11.5
13			3.5	

TABLE 4
NUMBER OF TIMES MARRIED

Women N = 120			Men N = 113		
1 time	62.5%	(75)	1 time	39%	(44)
2 times	21	(25)	2 times	29	(33)
3	12	(14)	3	15	(17)
4	2	(2)	4	11	(12)
5	2.5	(3)	5	2	(2)
6	1	(1)	6	3.5	(4)
			8	1	(1)
	100 %			100.5%	

virginity to escape a dreaded marriage, a desperate move in a country where even the appearance of illicit sex is a criminal offense. The meeting of a Muslim couple not married to each other in a secluded place (known as *khalwat*, or the crime of close proximity) is punishable by a stiff fine and a jail sentence, accompanied by notices in the newspapers of the couple's apprehension by the police. Other girls, less brave but equally stubborn, go through unwelcome marriage ceremonies but refuse conjugal relations, hoping to be quickly divorced.

When the marriage contract is signed, the groom must specify the amount of his payment to his bride (*mas kahwin*, or marriage gold). This may be as much as M$1,000 for a particularly desirable virgin bride or as little as M$1.00 for a previously married woman. Whatever the amount, it can either be paid to the bride at once or deferred to some future date. In case of divorce, any unpaid mas kahwin becomes part of the wife's settlement. She also has the right to keep any jewelry, whether brought into the marriage or purchased during its duration. Village women often perform their household tasks adorned with 22 carat gold earrings, bracelets, necklaces, and rings set with gems, although it is not uncommon for a bracelet to slip off a wrist and down a well,

[15]

Introaduction

necessitating a salvage operation and a ritual cleansing of the well
water. Women's jewels follow a seasonal cycle, disappearing into
the pawnshop during the monsoon season, when most income-
producing labor comes to a standstill, and emerging some months
later when the family has recouped its fortunes. Aside from its
function as a family nest egg, a piece of pawnable jewelry may
mean the difference between a divorced woman's proud independence and the humiliation of imposing a financial burden on
her kin. Women must be prepared to fend for themselves because, owing to the ease with which their husbands can obtain a
divorce, marriage offers no guarantee of long-term security.

Trengganu, which leads the country in the proportion of
Malays to other ethnic groups, also leads the country in the
proportion of divorces to marriages. In Trengganu, over a recent
ten-year period, divorces were 71.25 percent of all Muslim marriages (Gordon n.d.:16). Divorce is easy for a Malay man: he need
only pronounce the *talak* (I divorce thee) to dissolve the marriage.
He is not obliged to specify any grounds for his decision, and the
talak is valid whether it is pronounced as the result of long-
standing incompatibility or a momentary fit of anger. He must
then maintain his wife during her *iddah* period of three months.
If, during that time, the wife discovers she is pregnant, she is
entitled to be supported until her child has been delivered, at
which point her husband's obligation to her ceases. The bulk of
employment in Merchang is related to land, however only 22 percent of that land belongs to women. Many women lose access to
the land upon divorce and are obliged to work as hired hands
until they remarry, or to rely upon their parents for support.

About one-sixth of all divorces in Trengganu during the ten
years previously mentioned were subsequently revoked (Gordon
n.d.:16). This may take place during the iddah period after the
first or second talak, but if three talak have been pronounced,
over the course of many years or all at once, the marriage is

completely voided and cannot be resumed unless an intervening marriage (of the woman) has taken place. If the intervening marriage is entered into solely for the purpose of satisfying religious law, it is called a *cinabuta* marriage. In Malay this literally, and according to folk etymology, means "blind Chinese," but is actually derived from a Sanskrit word meaning "the divider" (Winstedt 1972*b*:73). The cinabuta groom, hired by the former husband, divorces the woman shortly after consummating the marriage. The original couple can marry after the wife's iddah period has been completed. Remarriage to a divorced wife who has had a hired interim husband is described by Malays as "licking what you have once spat out" (*sudah ludah lalu di jilat*). Two such cases were public knowledge in my parish, but the fact that the wives had submitted to other men's embraces caused so much embarrassment that neither of the couples was anxious to talk about it.

With this exception, there is no stigma attached to divorce and remarriage. The woman usually goes back to her parents' home with her children, to await her next marital episode. Although her ex-husband is under no financial obligation to his former wife after the *iddah* period, he is obliged to support his minor children. In many cases, however, the father defaults on his obligations. This may not work a hardship on those women who remarry quickly and bring their children into the new household, but for those few older women who remain unmarried and cannot depend on parental support, the economic consequences of divorce can be severe. Two of the poorest households in my area consisted of divorced wives in their forties and their children. In one case the father had moved to another state and had not been heard from in many years. In the other, the husband lived with his second wife not far from his former wife's home. They had a spacious house and a car, while the first wife and her two sons lived in a small and primitive structure. When the younger child became very ill, the father refused to pay for treatment and the mother had to depend on the charity of a bomoh, who treated the boy without fee.

It is possible for a Muslim woman to take the initiative in dissolving a marriage. She may offer her husband some material compensation, and surrender her claim to unpaid mas kahwin or iddah maintenance. She may also apply to the religious court for divorce by judicial decree on the grounds of impotence, insanity, a serious or repellent disease such as leprosy, or aggravated lack of maintenance. (Djamour 1966:77). In Trengganu, it is mandatory at the time of marriage for a husband to specify that his wife may obtain a divorce if he should abandon her or cause serious injury by beating her. Some women feel that occasional mild physical abuse is to be expected in marriage. To fight back is to run the risk of divorce. Although in case of injury or abandonment a wife can apply to the *kadzi* (Muslim registrar) for divorce, few village women invoke this law, as much from timidity as ignorance. When one woman in my village was advised to go to the kadzi to complain of aggravated lack of support, she said she would be too embarrassed and frightened to face him. All woman-instituted forms of divorce are extremely rare in Trengganu. According to the District Officer's records, from 1958– 1978 less than 3 percent of all divorces in Marang District, of which Merchang is a subdistrict, were instituted by women.

A wife may resort to making married life so miserable for her husband that she goads him into divorce. This domestic weapon may either be a knife which cuts the marriage bond cleanly, or a boomerang which leaves the wife in a worse position than she was before. I knew of cases where the husband became so bitter and vengeful that he disappeared from the village after pronouncing the talak without recording the divorce. The wife was left in limbo, with neither a husband nor a certificate of divorce that would permit her to marry another man.

Although a Muslim man is allowed to marry up to four wives at a time (women are limited to one husband), multiple marriage is quite rare in Merchang, particularly long-term multiple unions. Occasionally a man will satisfy his urge for sexual variety by marrying a second wife, tiring of her after several months, and divorcing her, while still keeping his first wife. A bomoh proudly told me that he never committed the serious sin of sleeping with women to whom he was not married. If he wanted them, he married them. Besides his first wife, to whom he had been married for twenty years, he had had six short-term wives. Aside from being considered moral behavior, short-term marriage does not carry the risk of arrest for khalwat.

The first wife is expected to be patient and forgiving. She usually consoles herself with the thought that her husband's affections have strayed because of love magic employed by the other woman. She may seek the help of a bomoh to apply counter-magic. Spells and procedures to compel love or produce hate, to return an erring husband to his wife, to break up an unsuitable attachment, or to cloud the eyes of a cuckolded husband are among the most lucrative of the bomoh's skills, and many laymen have also learned charms to help them in their love lives.

Some wives take matters into their own hands. Rather than rely upon secret retaliation through magic alone, they resort to open vilification of their rivals. One senior wife walked a mile each day to the home of her junior co-wife, a neighbor of mine, and stood outside her door, screaming imprecations. The embarrassed husband divorced the younger woman and went back to his old wife. She had taken a calculated risk, because the affair could have ended with her own divorce. People attributed her success not only to magic but to the fact that she was a wealthy woman in her own right, whereas the junior wife was a poor widow with several minor children.

Men and women are often thought to be faithful to their spouses because of *ilmu* (here, magical knowledge), especially if one of the partners is much older, ill favored or bad tempered. In

[19]

the rare cases of long-term multiple marriage, villagers are convinced that the man must possess a good deal of ilmu in order to be able to satisfy more than one wife, and to keep his wives from open warfare with one another. No Malay woman wants to share her husband with another woman, as much for economic reasons as for sexual pride. Men who have more than one wife must provide a separate household for each woman, preferably in separate villages. For a man who wants to marry double, ilmu is perhaps not as important as having some means of transportation. The two men in Merchang who had two wives apiece both had motorcycles. I knew of only one man in the area who currently had three wives—the taxicab owner in a neighboring parish.

Notwithstanding the ease of divorce, the final marriage is usually stable and long-lasting. I remember a conversation my husband had with a Malay man who boasted that the woman with whom he was presently living was his ninth wife. My husband asked him how long they had been married to each other. After a short discussion with his wife, he turned to my husband and, pointing to his wife, said, "This one has lasted about twenty-five years."

· 2 ·

Food: Belief and Behavior

Why should malnutrition exist in a land of eternal summer, where tropical fruits grow in profusion and every *padi* field abounds with fish? A good part of the problem, according to some commentators, lies in the failure of peasants to understand the relationship between what one eats and how one feels (for a discussion of this point see Foster and Anderson 1978:271–276). Rural Malays are said to undervalue many kinds of food because of mistaken dietary conceptions, and to remove foods from the diet, because of taboos, when, physiologically, they are most needed.

Malays are reported to believe that only two foods are worthy of the name: rice, which is essential for survival, and fish, which is necessary for strength (Wolff 1965). Vegetables are simply additives that improve the taste of rice, and fruits are "just pleasant things to keep the mouth busy" (1965:50). These ideas, Wolff believes, lead directly to extremely maladaptive behavior that culminates in malnutrition. Since deficiency diseases occur in a country rich in nutritious foods, "the observed deficiencies must be attributed to food habits" (1965:45). "In Malaya, it appears that people first should understand that vegetables are a food at all, before the Malays will readily accept the idea that a certain amount of vegetables is necessary in the diet" (1965:50). Wolff

[21]

adds that because "the Malay diet is monotonous, dietary imbalances are exaggerated" (1965:45).

Wolff's contentions appear to be supported by ethnographic evidence. Christine Wilson and Rosemary Firth report similar attitudes toward food in the east coast fishing communities in which they did their research. Wilson states that "vegetables are considered a relish not necessary to sustenance as are fish and rice" and adds that Peace Corps teachers told her that Malays on the east coast are "just [too] lazy to grow vegetable foods" (1970:140). Rosemary Firth surmises that "there does not seem to be any tradition that a fisherman's wife would do gardening on any scale" (Firth 1966:93), which Wilson amplifies to "nor . . . does there seem to be any tradition among *Malay* women to indulge in gardening" (Wilson 1970:140, emphasis supplied).

Malays in my parish conformed to the ideological pattern noted by Wolff. They did not consider fruits and vegetables necessary parts of a meal. "Fish and rice, rice and fish, that's us," one informant told me cheerfully. But theories feed on ideologies more surely than people do. Nourishment comes from what is actually eaten, whether or not this agrees with informants' statements about what constitutes a meal. While I found the food ideology exactly as it had been described in my reading, the behavior I encountered was far different.

WILD FOODS

I arrived in Merchang during the monsoon season, when high waves keep the fishermen ashore. I supposed the Malays' reported lack of interest in growing and eating vegetables would make them scarce in a community so far from a market. I expected to live on dried salted fish and rice until the rains abated. In fact, people were eating large quantities of dried fish and rice, and cultivated vegetables were unavailable, but I soon noticed people bringing home large bundles of greens daily. I was told

[22]

that these were *daun kayu*, a generic name for wild green vegetables, and that they formed a significant part of the diet, particularly during the rainy season.[1]

The complex ecology of Merchang provides the people with an extensive variety of cultivated and wild edible products.[2] Fruits and vegetables are widely cultivated and are available through most seasons of the year. The vast majority of villagers also know where to find and how to prepare wild foods. They are proud of their skills in locating and cooking daun kayu, and do not consider them fit only for emergency fare or the tables of the poor. City people also relish wild vegetables. At any time of the year at least fifteen wild varieties are sold in the city market of Kuala Trengganu, at prices comparable to those of cultivated plants. Even in the large markets of Kuala Lumpur, the nation's capital, at least six or seven wild species are offered for sale during much of the year. In Merchang, I counted seventy-two varieties of wild plants being consumed, as well as fifty-five varieties of cultivated fruits and vegetables.

Young shoots or leaves, sometimes of large trees, are plucked at all times of the year. Some are cooked, but many are eaten as salad (*ulam*), dipped into dried shrimp paste relish or added raw to rice or noodles. Some salad vegetables are never cooked, since they are thought to lose their *zat* (vitamins, goodness, essential nature) unless eaten raw. Wild vegetables can be found everywhere: *keladi agak*, which grows in the padi fields; *serian*, which prefers the secondary forest; many species of fern, found along the seashore; *terung pipit*, sweet little eggplants which grow wherever the soil is rich.

A favorite method of cooking vegetables, wild or cultivated, is *sayur* style, mixed with coconut cream, chilis, and fish. Palm cabbage, eaten raw or sayur style, is a welcome but infrequent addition to the diet, since it means the destruction of the tree. A particular delicacy is the *kulat sisir*, a mushroom that grows on dead rubber trees during the monsoon season.

[23]

The seeds of *buah jering*, *buah keredas*, and *buah petar* are gathered for local use and for sale. All are claimed to be palliatives for diabetes and, in fact, buah jering and buah petar are known to be diuretics, which could relieve the water retention common in diabetes. Jering, however, contains a volatile oil and an alkaloid that, if eaten in large quantities, inflames the kidneys and causes hematuria (Burkill 1966:1762). The Malays are aware of this danger, and to prevent it they boil jering in two or three changes of water, and keep them for a day before eating.

Three other wild vegetables require special treatment before they can be eaten, to avoid nausea, dizziness, and other toxic reactions. *Paku piah* must be boiled in at least three changes of water, *buah jeneris* is boiled twice and kept for two days before eating, and *buah berus* must have its outer skin scraped thoroughly before it is boiled in three changes of water. The time spent in its preparation, as well as its growing season (December–January, the height of the rainy season), make buah berus a food which is eaten only during the monsoon, when the sawmill closes down, the fishing boats are idle, and people have time to spare. The first monsoon season I spent in Merchang, large quantities of buah berus supplemented the dried fish and rice diet. During the second monsoon season there were shipments of fresh fish from the west coast and consumption of buah berus went down considerably.

Children can sometimes be prevailed upon to gather ulam growing near their homes, but collecting wild vegetables is usually the responsibility of adults, who often pluck them on their way back from work. Children never have to be coaxed to gather wild fruits. They are the principal consumers. Most wild fruits have a short season, so with the passing of the months the children's taste treats change. In February and March they hit wild mangosteens off the trees with long poles; from April through August they do the same to the sweet little red fruits of *kayu kelat*. January through May, children climb the *gucil* tree to pick its fruit; in July and August, it is the *sisek puyu*'s turn. Fruits that grow on bushes are easier to pick casually as the children pass by: the tiny tart red *buah binan setukar*, the sweet little white *buah gelam tikus*, the black *buah terajang*, yellow *buah ulat bulu*, and the *buah keduduk*, whose sweet blue fruits were once also used as ink.

Buah kemunting has small sweet red fruits year-round, but its peak season is October through December, when adults also gather large amounts to eat at home and to sell. Jungle fruits, such as *buah kelubi, buah salak* and *buah rekan*, are gathered extensively in season. In October and November large parties of children and adults spend whole days in the jungle collecting wild chestnuts, which they fry in a pan with clean sand.

CULTIVATED FOODS

Wild plants are available to all who care to gather them, but cultivated plants require work to grow or to purchase. Often families are obliged to do both. Although almost half the households in Merchang plant rice, the yield in recent years has been insufficient for any family's needs and has had to be supplemented by rice from Thailand or from the more productive states of Malaysia. Most of the crop is eaten by pests whose ravages, combined with unusually long dry seasons, make it "hardly worthwhile to plant padi," in the words of a kampung elder. But although the crop has been disastrous for at least five years, most people continue to plant year after year. This is partly because their rice lands, which are granted to them by the government, may be repossessed if they are not worked, and partly because of the wealth of myth and sentiment surrounding rice cultivation.

Magical ceremonies and precautions are no longer communal celebrations universally followed. Those who perform them do so privately, and their rites are considerably abbreviated in comparison with those described by Skeat (1972:218−249) and Wilkinson (1908:50). Before planting the rice, believers make four

[25]

small holes in the four corners of the field and bury plants of magical significance: *daun sepulih*, used because its name means return to health; *daun buluh gading*, whose golden color provides a sympathetic impetus to the rice to mature healthy and yellow instead of diseased and rusty red, and whose name makes it a magical defense against the *ulat gading*, an insect that makes its cocoon inside the rice stems; *daun pinang* and *daun geribu seni*, the former a component of spirit offerings and the latter used to tie them; and pineapple leaves, whose spiny spikes are said to frighten the spirits who afflict women in childbirth. The field of rice is often compared to a pregnant woman, and the harvest climaxes in the taking of the Rice Baby, a stalk of rice which is swaddled like a human child. The harvested rice is stored in a special bin with a coconut, coconut oil, limes, beluru root, bananas, sugar cane, water, and a comb, all for the use of the Rice Spirit (*semangat padi*), personified as a timid young girl (see also Firth 1974:192−195). Since she is easily frightened, the rice must be brought back to the storeroom to the accompaniment of lullabies and left there in silence for three days. Those who still practice traditional harvest rituals complain that modern methods of rice production frighten the Rice Spirit from the fields. There is less rice to eat than there used to be, they say, and it doesn't fill your belly as it should.

Many people think that the decline in local rice production would not have come about without a breakdown in traditional practices and a lack of community solidarity. In the past, all the rice growers hired one bomoh (magical-medical practitioner) to banish wild pigs, rodents, worms, and other vermin from their fields. Recently there has been a demographic change: many people from Kelantan, where land pressure is intense, have migrated to Merchang, settling in previously unpopulated areas and cutting down the jungle under the supervision of their own bomoh. There is no longer any consensus regarding which ritual practitioner should treat the fields. Some people, responding to a

[26]

general increase in Islamic orthodoxy in Malaysia, have substituted Arabic prayers for the bomoh's spells; others are skeptical about the need for any supernatural intervention whatsoever in the growing of rice. This spectrum of belief has produced what older villagers call "a confusion" which they say is responsible for the failure of the rice crop. Others ascribe it to the will of God.

Religion enters the picture in another way as well. As more people move into the area and the jungle is cut down, there are fewer natural checks on vermin. As the tigers' habitat shrinks and many are shot when they wander into human territory, the number of wild pigs who had been the tigers' prey has increased tremendously. In parts of the Philippines, similar conditions have proved a bonanza to the Agta negritoes, who hunt the now easily available pigs and gladly eat wild pork (Peterson 1977). Since pig flesh is forbidden to Muslims, the growing porcine population, rather than adding to the Malays' diet, causes a deficit by destroying their crops.

As human habitation moves closer to the padi fields, the wild civet cats and monitor lizards, previously welcome because they keep the rodent population down, have themselves become vermin because they raid the chicken coops. Householders kill them at sight, ridding their poultry of enemies and their rice fields of friends.

Among the many varieties of vegetables cultivated in Merchang are some—like green beans, cabbage, pumpkin, eggplant, tomato, mustard greens, and peanuts—which are well known in America. Tiny baby ears of corn are boiled and eaten cob and all. Less familiar are the bottle gourd and *kangkong* (*Ipomoea reptans*), a green leafy plant something like spinach. The chili pepper, originally a native of America, is now an indispensable part of Malay cookery, grown even by those who plant only small kitchen gardens.

Cassava, another native of America, is grown extensively, both for its root and its leaves. Its ability to remain indefinitely in the

[27]

soil without rotting, the exuberance with which it grows, and the little care it demands make it a popular snack and an occasional substitute for rice in poorer homes, but people do not value it as highly as rice either for its taste or its power to sustain health and life. Malays remember the Japanese occupation as the time they were forced to eat cassava while their conquerors filled up on rice. Deprived of an important source of nutrients, Malays became weak and lost their resistance to infectious diseases. Cassava root fills the belly but slights the tissues, since it yields approximately the same amount of calories as rice but provides only one-tenth as much protein and a fraction of the B vitamins. When yeast is added and cassava root is allowed to ferment, it becomes *tapai*, a mildly alcoholic treat served especially at Hari Raya Puasa, the festival following Ramadan, the month of fasting. Although Islam forbids drinking alcoholic beverages, the rules, as interpreted by east coast Malays, do not prohibit eating alcoholic foods.

Sweet potatoes, taro, and several varieties of potato do not take the place of rice but are served with the rice meal as side dishes, or later, as snacks. Many types of unripe fruit are eaten sayur style: cooked this way, papaya, watermelon, and two kinds of jackfruit, as well as the male flower of the banana plant and the skins of *buah setar*, *buah setial*, and *buah jentik*, are popular accompaniments to the rice meal. The yellow fruit of the cashew tree can double as a stewed vegetable. It may also be eaten raw, if one is careful to keep its copious juices from leaving bright blue stains on one's clothing. Its leaves are eaten as salad, and its nut, which is produced at the end of the fruit rather than within, is roasted to remove toxicity.

Dozens of different kinds of bananas and plantains are grown in Merchang. So are papayas, mangosteens, star fruit, soursops, sapodillas, pineapple, limes, rambutan (*Nephelium lappaceum*), so-called because of its hairy-looking skin (*rambut* means hair), rambai (*Baccauea motleyana*), langsat and duku (two types of *Sansium domesticum*), small tan fruits with a grapefruitlike taste, four

[28]

kinds of mango, and four of guava. Two varieties of jackfruit produce enormous fruits—specimens three feet long are quite common. The fruit is protected when half ripe by a burlap bag, and ants are encouraged to swarm over it to protect it from other insects. Durian is not grown extensively in Merchang, but its taste is so highly prized that people are willing to travel twenty miles and more for this luscious spiky fruit. Devotees of durian (among them, the tiger) grow so fond of the fruit that its noxious smell becomes perfume to them, a harbinger of the delights to be found inside its hard spiny shell. The large seeds of durian and jack-fruit, boiled, taste like chestnuts. Coconuts are a frequent ingredient in Malay dishes. Macaques are trained to pluck the mature nuts from the palms—they become flustered when required to pick a young fruit. The flesh of immature coconuts has a jellylike consistency and can easily be scooped out and mixed with its own water and some sugar for a refreshing drink.

IDEOLOGY AND BEHAVIOR

If the rich profusion of fruits and vegetables cultivated and gathered wild in Merchang appears to conflict with Malay dietary conceptions as reported by Wolff and other researchers, and by Malays themselves, the quantities consumed present an even more striking example of the differences between stated ideology and perceived behavior.

Although Wolff (1965) suggests that, to a Malay, fruits are an unimportant part of the diet, "something to keep the mouth busy," in Merchang, during peak seasons, fruit forms a substantial part of many meals. Besides the unripe fruits served as side dishes, ripe pineapple and watermelon were often eaten with rice. Pregnant women in particular craved fruit and sometimes made a meal of bread and fruit alone when the taste and smell of fish had begun to pall.

It is true that in Merchang vegetables are thought of as a relish,

[29]

not absolutely essential for survival or strength. The portions consumed, however, are considerably larger than we might expect from a food in the relish category: 40 to 230 grams per meal. According to data supplied by the U.S. Agricultural Research Service (U.S. Department of Agriculture 1978), the average weight of a day's intake of green beans by an American adult is 69.4 grams, that of peas 81. So the portions consumed in Merchang as a relish are comparable to an average American serving of a vegetable.

A further comparison of American and Malay food ideologies and behaviors yields another interesting insight. The Committee on Food Habits of the U.S. National Research Council (1943) reported that although in all ethnic groups and income levels they surveyed vegetables was the food category most frequently cited as essential to the diet, a survey of Ohio farm families revealed that only 34 percent of the adults and 37 percent of the children ate at least one green or yellow vegetable daily. In contrast, although Malay ideology rates vegetables low in the food hierarchy, 63.5 percent of all households I surveyed ate a green or yellow vegetable at least once a day, and 35 percent twice a day. The differences between expressed belief and actual behavior are striking in both instances.

Since it is clear that in an ecologically rich zone food ideology does not lead automatically to unwise eating patterns that produce nutritional disorders, how can we explain the dietary deficiencies that Wolff attributes to Malay food ideology? The survey he cites to support his claim of "widely observed deficiency of foodstuffs containing vitamin A" in the Malay diet was taken in an inland district of Perak, known to contain a high proportion of malnourished children (Thomson 1960). The most serious problem Thomson noted was protein malnutrition. The reasons she gave for health problems in this area include:

1. Ecological considerations: fish were not plentiful in the area and, although a small amount of fresh sea fish was available,

[30]

it was expensive, since it had to be imported from the coast, a distance of seventy-six miles.

2. Economic considerations: underemployment, resulting in incomes too low to provide an adequate diet.

3. Health problems: widespread infestation of nematodes. All toddlers examined had heavy loads of *Ascaris lumbricoides* and diarrhea was frequent. Frequent attacks of diarrhea can precipitate the onset of kwashiorkor in an already malnourished child.

With these and several other more minor problems to choose from, it is hard to explain why Wolff emphasized the "meanings of food" to the exclusion of other factors. Thomson mentions customs affecting diet only as a factor that may combine with others to produce ill health.

Emphasis on dietary beliefs has had an unfortunate impact on health programs in the Third World which, too often, have centered on efforts to educate mothers, on the assumption that changing their beliefs would lead to good nutritional health for their families (e.g., Cravioto 1958; Perez et al. 1969). For example, although most of the rural Mexican children who develop severe cases of malnutrition come from the poorest segments of society, attempts to improve their diet tend to call particular attention to their mothers' beliefs about "hot" and "cold" foods (for a critique of these programs see DeWalt, Kelly and Pelto 1980:206).[3] The children of wealthier neighbors, who share the same humoral concepts, are healthy despite their mothers' beliefs. As Thomson's study shows, beliefs that further deplete an already marginal diet can contribute to malnutrition, but the circumstances responsible for the marginal diet must still remain the paramount cause.

Attributing the monotony of the Malay diet to a faulty belief system, and linking this lack of variety to malnutrition, represents both an overestimation of the strength of other people's culture-bound concepts and a lack of recognition of our own.

To criticize something as monotonous implies a positive evalu-

[31]

ation of novelty and change characteristic of our own society. People in other societies do not necessarily think of repetition as boring, but may find it, rather, comforting, assuring them that what is known and understood will not suddenly change. Malays do not think of rice meals as monotonous. Rice is satisfying, necessary, the staff of life. They would not consider alternating rice with corn, bread, and potatoes to be an improvement.

Wolff points to the monotony of the Malay diet as an exacerbating factor in dietary imbalance, but this is not a nutritional axiom. Although nutritionists recommend a varied diet, they know that good health can be associated with a diet that is considerably more limited than that of rural Malays.

The most extreme example of which I am aware is that of the El Molo tribe who live on the shores of Lake Rudolph in Kenya. Fish is their basic diet, supplemented infrequently by seabirds, a crocodile, or a hippopotamus. Nevertheless, physical examinations of these people revealed the El Molo to be generally well nourished (Brown et al. 1966). Although it was expected that this limited diet would lead, at the very least, to vitamin C deficiency, neither clinical nor biochemical tests supported this expectation (Hansen et al. 1966).

The diet in Merchang is infinitely more varied than that of the El Molo. Within a seven day period, one woman (by no means wealthy) ate, aside from the ever-present rice, four kinds of cake, two types of cracker, and some wheat rolls. She had seven species of fish prepared five different styles, and a stew of clams and vegetables. She ate six different types of vegetables and seven varieties of fruit. This diet, consumed during September, a time of abundance of fruits and vegetables, is typical for the season. Only a contemporary American city dweller, living within reach of a giant supermarket with its enormous range of foods and ability to secure products from afar which are out of season locally, could call such a diet "monotonous."

[32]

DIET AND ECOLOGY

The picture I have presented of the bewildering variety of edible plants eaten in Merchang (a total of 127 different kinds) contrasts vividly with Wilson's description of the Malay diet. We appear to be discussing two populations separated by oceans or miles of terrain, rather than two groups of east coast Malays living only twelve miles apart. Yet demographic and ecological differences between Merchang and RuMuda (Wilson's research site) can account for these differences. Both Wilson and Firth lived in seaside fishing communities, where the sandy soils are not conducive to agriculture. The failure of Malay fishermen and their wives to grow vegetables does not reside in their laziness or lack of gardening traditions, but rather in the unprofitability of this activity in their ecological zone. The inhabitants of RuMuda have settled near the beaches and have not penetrated deeply inland. One would expect to find few wild fruits and vegetables thriving within easy reach, and that, in fact, is the case. Residents of RuMuda would have to travel far from their homes to collect daun kayu. In Merchang, wild fruits and vegetables are collected opportunistically on a daily basis, and parties rarely form for large-scale exploitation of edible jungle resources. Were one to assume that a similar pattern would prevail in RuMuda, one would not expect wild plants to form any significant part of the diet, a hypothesis that is borne out by Wilson's observations (1970:139).

The danger in any community study is that data may be generalized to cover larger populations and areas that might be different from the smaller unit. Data from Wilson's, Firth's, and other studies have been used to characterize the eating habits of all Malays rather than to illustrate dietary behavior only in a certain type of ecological zone. The differences between the eating patterns of the residents of RuMuda and those of Mer-

[33]

chang point out the need for microecological studies and provide a caveat to those who too easily make generalizations, whether about ecology, diet, or any other sphere affecting human existence and behavior.

Although anthropologists, who often spend extended periods of time exploring a culture in depth, must guard against generalizing from the particular, nutritionists must be wary of not examining the particular sufficiently.

There are many pitfalls into which nutritional surveys may fall. They face serious drawbacks, since they are typically short-term investigations that rely primarily upon asking questions rather than observing behavior: (1) the diet changes during the year, so catching the diet at any one time will give a false impression of the whole; and (2) a short-term investigator may not know what kinds of questions will be successful in unearthing the data one seeks, since one is unlikely to be conversant with the local dialect and customs. For example, asking villagers in Merchang how many times a week they eat sayur (which simply means vegetables in standard Malay) may evoke a response in terms of cultivated vegetables only, or in terms of fruits and vegetables prepared sayur style. It will not ordinarily evoke an answer that also covers ulam (raw or cultivated vegetables eaten as salad), or daun kayu (the generic name for wild greens). Data obtained in this manner will yield a false picture of the actual diet.

These problems—the confusion of the general and the particular, emphasis on ideological rather than ecological and economic bases for malnutrition, the presumed leap from belief to action, and the nature of belief—will recur as I discuss the Malay humoral system, and the reproductive cycle in Merchang.

· 3 ·

The Malay Humoral System and the Concept of Bisa

The Malays, in common with people from many past and present cultures, categorize foods, diseases, and treatments according to intrinsic qualities, which they refer to as "heating" or "cooling." Although temperature may be one consideration (e.g., using a fire to heat the beds of women in the puerperium), they are not equivalent to thermal measurements. In the Malay system, humoral qualities of foods are not changed by altering their temperature. Thus, squash boiling on the stove is still humorally "very cold," while alcohol, even if iced, is still "extremely hot." Since illness is thought to occur when the equilibrium of these opposing elements is disturbed, the practical application of this theory aims at restoration of the body's balance, using foods and treatments that decrease the element in excess and/or increase the deficient humor.

HUMORAL PATHOLOGY

Humoral pathology, versions of which are found in Arabic, Chinese, and Indian Ayurvedic medicine, was part of European medical tradition from before the time of Hippocrates until well

[35]

into the seventeenth century A.D. Malaya, an early trading center for travelers from China[1] and India, exchanged medical ideas as well as goods with representatives of these cultures, and received a further injection of humoral theory when Arabic medicine came to Southeast Asia along with Islam.

Here the humoral system may have found ready acceptance because it shares a point of resemblance with beliefs of Malayan aborigines centering around childbirth. Their food avoidances are found primarily within the context of pregnancy and the puerperium. After delivery, restrictions are imposed on the mother's diet which may last from ten days in some groups and until the baby begins to walk in others (Skeat and Blagden 1906; Bolton 1972; for a discussion of food restrictions among the Semai see Dentan 1965). Sakai (Blandas) mothers are forbidden to drink or wash in cold water for ten days following delivery (Skeat and Blagden 1906:II, 10). This practice has a direct counterpart in the Malay system, which assumes a new mother is in a cold state that must be treated by prescribing warm substances and proscribing cold. The practice of "roasting" the new mother over or beside a fire, common throughout Southeast Asia (Hart, Rajadhon and Coughlin 1965) and observed by aboriginal peoples of Malaya as well as by Muslim Malays (Skeat and Blagden 1906:II, 2), is also consonant with the tenets of humoral pathology.

Outside observers have generally considered contemporary humoral systems to be symbolic, or magical, and have explained them in psychological or sociological terms. Burgess and Dean (1962:68) believe giving "heating" and "cooling" foods is a magical attempt to evade or appease an apparently external threat that is actually a projection of internal stresses. A similar view is taken by Currier, who considers this type of system a model of social relations, that is, the ideal of balance within the human body echoes the ideal of balance within the social body, and fear of "cold" diseases is an extension of the child's loss of maternal

[36]

warmth during weaning (Currier 1966:251).

In contrast, those who believe in the reality of humoral distinctions perceive them as having an empirical basis. The ultimate criterion informants give for determining whether a substance is "hot" or "cold" is its effect on their bodies. Orso (1970:49) found that when a Costa Rican's experience disagreed with a learned classification, the classification of that substance changed for that individual. Harwood (1971) remarked on this tendency among Puerto Ricans. When South Indians were asked how they would determine the correct category for a new food, they said they would have to eat it for several days to see whether it had heating or cooling affects on their own bodies (Beck 1969:571). In a study largely devoted to the symbolic aspects of shamanistic curing in Mexico, Fabrega and Silver (1973:86) state that humoral beliefs and practices "are virtually the only place in Zinacanteco medicine where notions of cause and effect involving bodily events and processes are linked in a clear and specific manner to illness and to the action of remedies." Despite this strongly empirical aspect of humoral pathology, few investigators have examined the system for possible insights into human ecology (Logan 1972, McCullough 1973, and Lindenbaum 1977 are notable exceptions). Instead, most have criticized it as a barrier to acceptance of hospital-based medicine and as a contributor to ill health, particularly malnutrition (for the Malay case see Siti Hasmah 1968; Chen 1972, 1973, 1974—1975; Wilson 1970, 1971, 1973; Wilson et al. 1970; Millis 1958).[2]

VARIABILITY AND THE INDIVIDUAL

Although anthropologists should be as attentive to variability as they are to consensus within a population, investigators of humoral systems have been disturbed by their informants' lack of agreement in categorizing food items. In the same community, some people classify an item as "cold" while others call it neutral

[37]

or "hot." Discussions of humoral systems often feature extensive food lists, some merely indicating into which (occasionally contradictory) categories a particular food has been placed (e.g., Hart 1969:79−89), while others show the number of respondents who classified each food differently (e.g., Wilson 1970: 286−290). These apparent inconsistencies have been attributed to differing family traditions (Wilson 1970:286), and have been said to lack any systematic basis (Burgess and Dean 1962:34). The problem, however, is created by the investigators' expectations of finding a taxonomy with clear-cut boundaries, a classificatory system in which categories are forever frozen like flies in amber.

Humoral systems are dynamic rather than taxonomic. They not only admit the possibility of variation, they incorporate it into the model.[3] Variability within a system is a hallmark of Malay belief about the essential nature of life. Humoral—and all other beliefs—are subject to alteration and interpretation. Not only are individuals considered to be different from one another physically and temperamentally but also are assumed to change as they pass through the stages of life, seasons of the year, and hours of the day.

The bodies of babies and young children are considered to be colder than those of adults. A proof of this lies in the youngsters' greater tendency to have (generally cold) stomachaches. Healthy adult bodies are neither hot (*panas*) nor cold (*sejuk*), but *sederhana* (glossed as "the proper mean" in Wilkinson 1959:II, 1033). Within this norm, women are slightly cooler and men slightly warmer. Old people return to the beginning of the cycle and become colder than normal adults, evidenced by "cold" rheumatic pains.

Just as people are colder in the morning and evening of their lives, so, too, are they colder in the beginning and end of each day. Thus, it is considered safer to eat "cooling" foods during late morning, afternoon, and evening than in the early morning or at night. Conversely, if one is taking "hot" medicine, it is wise to take

[38]

smaller doses around noon so that the essential humoral balance will not be disturbed.

A person's humoral circumstances are also governed by the seasons of the year. On the east coast of Malaysia there are three seasons: the monsoon (known as *musim banjir*, the season of floods, and *musim sejuk*, the cold season), the extremely hot, dry season (*musim kemarau*, the season of drought), and the months between the two extremes, a period not given a name. During the dry season when the weather is sometimes unbearably hot, people eat extremely cold foods which they avoid during cooler months. In the chilly monsoon season the diet is reduced to dried salted fish (a hot food) and rice (sederhana), with the addition of whatever wild vegetables one is able to gather. High winds and torrential rains make it impossible for fishermen to take their boats out, and few cultivated vegetables are available. None of the wild vegetables falls into the extremely cold category: some are considered neutral while others are even hot. Nature, it seems, has made available only foods that will not intensify the unpleasant coldness of the rainy season, so that foolish people, craving "very cold" foods like gourd or papaya, do not have the opportunity of indulging in such harmful practices.

When I first arrived in Trengganu, my neighbors assumed that, since I came from a cold climate, my body would need vast quantities of "hot" beefsteak to function properly. Rural Malays rarely eat beef, but during the days of British Malaya they had become aware of the British predilection for beef, which they interpreted humorally. When my first dry season arrived, my assistant suggested I cut down on meat and eat a lot of cooling fruits and vegetables. Otherwise, he feared, my body, unused to the heat of the tropics, would quickly dehydrate.

The importance of balance and the dynamic nature of the system are shown by distinguishing its marked and unmarked features.[4] Between the extremes of hot and cold a neutral category designates the proper mean. This is an unmarked category,

[39]

the most common and least problematic within the system. Of the ages of man, the one that lasts longest and is considered healthiest is also the one that does not have to be specified linguistically. *Orang*, the general term for human being, can be used without modifiers for those who have passed childhood but have not yet attained old age. Children are referred to as *budak*, while old people are called *orang tua*. The least problematic and longest time of the year has no inclusive name whatsoever, while the extremes of cold and wet, hot and dry are named. The marked features are specially attended to in action as well as language.

THE BODILY HUMORS

An integral part of the Malay humoral system is that of complementary body fluids. Blood is conceived of as the "hot" humor, while phlegm (*lendir*) is the "cold." Lendir includes substances Westerners consider quite diverse; the organizing principle is that of sliminess: the mucus of a runny nose, lymph, semen, egg whites, the viscous matter in okra, certain bananas and other "slimy" fruits and vegetables, and the slime on the skin of certain fish.

Since it is a cold element, lendir can coagulate within the human body. A *tongkol berlendir* (lump of phlegm) is the Malay term for what we call a knotted muscle. Clotting can be helpful: lendir acts like cement to mend broken bones. However, when it forms clots it causes pain which some lay people call "a spirit eating at you." In contrast, bomoh explain that the pain is caused by a clot of lendir which stops the flow of blood through the veins. When blood does not flow normally through an area, it becomes cold, and muscles move from their true places.[5] This can result in leg aches, backache, or even pain and paralysis of muscles controlling facial expression (this seems to be Bell's Palsy, which responds to massage, the Malay treatment of preference), Mas-

[40]

sage breaks up the clots of lendir, allowing the blood to flow freely.

Malays consider blood so hot that it cannot clot within the body, though it can when it comes into contact with cold air. Changes in body temperature, however, can affect the speed of blood flow. A hot illness produces a rapid pulse and a cold condition a slow pulse, since cold thickens the blood. Some people develop abnormally hot blood, either because of an illness that causes the blood to become dirty (for instance *sembap*, characterized by edema) or because of *darah tinggi* (literally, high blood). Since overheated blood is thought to rush to the head, considered normally hotter than the rest of the body, causing dimmed vision, headache, dizziness, and faintness, it may be possible to ease this condition by draining off some of the dirty or excess blood by means of cupping. Since bloodletting does, in fact, temporarily relieve the symptoms of severe hypertension[6] (and was the treatment of preference in Western medicine until modern times), the success of the therapy reinforces belief in the humoral system (cf. Harwood 1971:1156).[7]

In similar humoral systems in Latin America, pregnant women are believed to be hotter than normal (Fabrega 1974:239). This concept is the antithesis of Malay belief concerning conception and gestation. Beliefs about the postpartum period, however, are similar in all humoral systems of which I am aware: after childbirth a woman enters a "cold" state because her body has been depleted of blood, the "hot" body fluid. This postpartum "cold" state is physiological as well as symbolic. The fact that this physiologically cold period lasts for only a fraction of the forty day postpartum period is no more prejudicial to belief in the humoral system than the fact that bloodletting only relieves hypertension temporarily. Immediate empirical observations suffice to support the symbolic logic of the humoral system by giving "proof" of its validity.

THE HUMORS AND DIET

Like adherents of humoral systems in other cultures, Malays claim they observe their own bodies to resolve questions about categorizing foods. In a survey which I conducted in two hamlets in the parish, thirty-eight people, or 62 percent of my respondents, said they could feel the effects of eating "hot" and "cold" foods. Twenty-five percent, or fifteen individuals, said they themselves could feel only extremes of humoral temperature and relied on older or more sensitive people to judge less obvious foods. Thirteen percent, or eight individuals, said they never concerned themselves with such matters since they were exceptionally healthy no matter what they ate, and one added that, as far as he was concerned, hot coffee was hot, ice was cold, and humoral beliefs were nonsense.[8]

I postponed this survey for more than a year, since I was convinced that simply asking people how they would classify individual food items would yield the usual mystifying, contradictory charts. I hoped, rather, to be able to formulate questions that might uncover the thought processes and criteria Malays use. I had already collected a good deal of food-related data, and now added to this information by having long discussions with three key informants. I conferred with them separately, asking about individual foods and searching for possible organizing principles. They had never before had any reason to think analytically about this topic, but they were quick to agree or disagree with my tries at formulations. The questions I eventually used were phrased with their help.

Some questions grew out of comments about foods in particular situations. For example, I was present at many births and often heard women discussing which foods were advisable and which inadvisable after delivery. Coffee was all right because it was hot, tea was not since it was cold. What was the difference between these two beverages, both served thermally hot? That

[42]

was simple, I was told. Coffee is bitter and tea is *kelat*.[9] By listing all bitter and all kelat foods and inquiring about each one's humoral qualities, I discovered that everything bitter is hot and everything kelat is cold.

Other questions were derived from humoral comments not associated with foods. When one of my neighbors gashed his leg, he was taken to the seaside to bathe it. The "heat" of the water would dry up the blood, I was told. What is there about seawater that makes it hotter than regular water? The salt, of course. Are the fish that live in the sea hot? No, they are sederhana (the proper mean), but if you add salt and dry them they become hot.

Still other questions arose from those positions in which key informants placed certain foods along a hot-cold continuum. Some of the groupings appeared to have an obvious relationship while others were incomprehensible. Of the first sort, fats and fatty foods had been grouped as hot. But what did beans, cucumbers, gourds, and sweet potatoes have in common? To me the connection was unclear, to my informants it was obvious—they are all creepers and climbers (*berjalar*).

All agreed, moreover, that while most bananas were sederhana, some were definitely cold. Was it because some are eaten raw while others are cooked? No, I was told, it was because some are berlendir (slimy). This, then, helped to explain why okra and other viscous plants are classified as cold.

Some of my attempted formulations were rejected, that is, orange or yellow plants are hotter than green plants; roots and tubers growing away from sunlight are colder than leaves and fruits exposed to the sun.

The questions employed in the survey were phrased neutrally: Are bitter foods hot, cold, or sederhana? They contained both questions derived in the above manner and others invented by me as checks (such as "Are wild plants hot, cold or sederhana?"). The differences in response to the agreed-upon questions and the checks were striking—all agreed that salt and salty fish were hot, the majority (82%) agreed that creepers and climbers were cold, that viscous foods are cold (68%) and bitter foods hot (68%). In contrast, only 8 percent said that all fruits are cold and none believed that all wild plants could be placed en masse in any category. When confronted by a noncategory (i.e., wild plants, or all plants that do not creep or climb), people usually insisted on explaining that some of the items were hot while others were cold.

Besides asking about groups, I asked about individual items. Explanations were often volunteered when foods that conceptually should have been in one category appeared in another; if not offered, they were elicited. My final questions were "How do you know whether foods are hot, cold or sederhana? What happens if a healthy person eats a lot of hot foods; if a sick person does? What happens if a healthy person eats a lot of cold foods; if a sick person does? Does mixing hot and cold foods change their qualities; does cooking?"

Here are the results:

"Hot" Foods

1. Fats, both animal and vegetable, are considered hot because they satiate the appetite quickly and give the eater a feeling of well-being.[10] Durian, which has a higher fat content than any other fruit (except avocado, unknown on the east coast of Malaysia), is considered extremely hot. Malays claim that overeating durian can produce fever in susceptible individuals. I, myself, felt warm after eating durian, possibly for a reason unknown to my informants. Studies at the Institute for Medical Research in Kuala Lumpur show that durian's final chemical breakdown products are similar to those of alcohol (Wilson 1970:48).

2. Alcohol is hot. Although Islamic religious law forbids alcoholic beverages, Malays eat a mildly alcoholic dish called *tapai*, made from either fermented cassava root or glutinous rice prepared with yeast. Tapai is considered very hot.

3. Spices in general are hot. Malays have one term for thermal and humoral heat (*panas*) and another for spiciness (*pedas*). Spices are both pedas and panas since eating them produces heat in the mouth and perspiration on the skin, physiological proof of humoral doctrine.

4. Animal proteins, including eggs and milk but excluding fresh fish, are hot.[11] Like fats, they produce satiety and well-being. However, the categorization of milk as hot is also backed up by humoral logic. If milk were cold it would give babies, whose bodies are colder than those of adults, stomachache (a cold ailment). Since milk is good for babies it must be at least warm.

5. Salty foods are hot. The designation applies to dried salted fish, one of the mainstays of the diet. It also refers by extension, to plants that grow near the seaside and become hot because of the influence of the salty sea. One criterion for inclusion in this category is the effect of salty foods on people who have abnormally hot blood; they suffer headache, dizziness, and dimmed vision—all symptoms of excessive heat rising to the head. Another criterion is the association with salty blood, the hot body fluid.

6. Bitter foods are hot. The rationale appears to rest on two major considerations. First, a bitter wild herb (*lapeng budak—Clerodendron* sp. Fam. Verbenaceae) is used as the sovereign remedy for constipation. Malays believe the herb's "heat" softens hard stool. Second, an infusion of bitter roots (*akar kayu*) is an important part of the Malay pharmacopoeia, used as a general tonic and especially important for women during the reproductive cycle. Most new mothers drink akar kayu since it is believed to restore body heat depleted during delivery by blood loss. Pregnant women avoid akar kayu, since heat is considered antithetical to the fetus. Following the same reasoning, women who are trying to abort may drink akar kayu. If a particular vegetable is bitter at one stage in its growth it is hot during that stage, but not necessarily at any other. The same particularity applies to parts of

[45]

plants: only those parts that taste bitter are hot. The rest of the plant may be categorized differently.

"Cold" Foods

1. Juicy fruits and vegetables are cold, as are fruits and vegetables that need a great deal of water for growth. The rationale is the close relationship of wet to cold. This is seen more clearly in the case of jungle vegetation, also usually classified as cold. Contrary to the expectations of those who have never experienced jungle ambiance, the exudation of the rain forest is cool and wet.

2. Fruits and vegetables such as okra and certain varieties of plantain that exude viscous matter (lendir) are cold by association with phlegm (lendir), the cold body humor.

3. Sour fruits and vegetables are thought to be cold because many pregnant women crave sour foods and eat them without harm. Malays reason that if these foods were hot they would precipitate abortions since everything the mother eats finds its way to the fetus.

4. Plants that taste kelat are cold. Tea is cold while coffee, which is bitter, is hot. Several types of leaves used for fever-lowering poultices are kelat themselves or come from a plant whose fruit is kelat. Classification of these plants as cold rests on their ability to relieve a hot illness.

5. Vines, creepers, and climbers are cold. Although the Malay language does not include rules for gender, Malays categorize some natural objects, such as anthills, dew, brine, and gravel as male or female, the big, tall, or pointed being male while the short, squat, or clinging are female. As "feminine" plants, vines and creepers partake of the naturally cooler female quality.

When I asked people to classify individual items, most stayed close to these patterns. For the minority who relied on other people's classifications, variation may well be a function of informal education based on differing family traditions, for example, someone whose mother classified a food in an unexpected category because it gave her digestive problems may continue to classify that food the same way, even though it did not produce that effect on him. The usual reason, however, for classifying an item in an unexpected category was its effect on the person doing the classifying. For instance, one man told me that although everyone else said lapeng budak is hot since it relieves constipation, he would not classify it as hot since it did not produce the same result for him. By the same token, although the majority classified taro as cold, people who could eat large amounts without getting stomachache classified it as neutral (sederhana).

Neutral (Unmarked) Foods

Less than a quarter of my informants classified foods only as hot or cold. The rest recognized a sometimes extensive category which, for them, was neutral (sederhana, the proper mean). Sederhana foods can be eaten with no danger. Even for most who recognized only a simple dichotomy, two items—rice and fresh fish—stood outside the humoral system, neither hot nor cold. Within the domain of food they are unmarked.

Malays conceive of their foods hierarchically: rice is necessary for survival, animal proteins (for all practical purposes, fish) are necessary for strength, vegetables are simply additives to improve the taste of rice, and fruits are "pleasant things to keep the mouth busy" (Wolff 1965:50). The only items considered essential are rice and fish. The Malay gloss for "to eat a meal" is *makan nasi* (literally, to eat rice). Even when people knew that my breakfast had consisted of coffee and wheat cakes, they referred to the meal as makan nasi. *Lauk*, the generic term for side dishes served with rice, is also used, unmodified, to mean fish. In some parts of Malaysia, the cry of the fish-seller is "Lauk." (Wilkinson 1959,II: 661). My language teacher in Kuala Lumpur translated *lauk* as "the fish that is served with rice." I learned later that the term can cover a multitude of other items, with appropriate modifications.

Hot and cold foods, the marked features of this domain, are considered nonessential to the daily diet. They may injure some people's health consistently and, even in the case of normal people with transient illnesses, must occasionally be cut out of the diet or eaten in reduced quantities. Marked themselves, they are associated with marked features in another domain. Good health, assumed to be present unless otherwise specified, is unmarked, while deviations are marked. Rice is never removed from the diet. Sick people are encouraged to eat rice and, indeed, a sign of returning health is an improvement in appetite sufficient for the patient to consume the large plate of rice most Malays eat at least twice daily. Fish soup is considered very strengthening for invalids. Classifying rice and fresh fish as either hot or cold would be destructive to the internal logic of Malay belief, as well as to health.

Regulating the Daily Diet

Although most Malays have definite ideas about the intrinsic heat of their daily food, few actually regulate their diets on humoral principles. Normal adults whose bodies are balanced between humoral extremes do not have to concern themselves with dietary adjustments. With few exceptions, people said that mixing hot and cold foods will produce the proper mean. They do not, however, refer to this concept as a guiding force when choosing foods. They feel that simply eating a normal diet will ensure proper humoral balance, but if balance is lacking in a given meal most people will still experience no difficulty. On the whole, it is only those whose bodies congenitally deviate from the norm who eliminate or cut down on foods in their daily diets. Markedness in the humoral system is bipolar. A person who is already unbalanced toward either polarity will be wary of eating foods that will cause further imbalance.

Most people I questioned agreed that some individuals experience digestive problems when they eat large amounts of cold foods. Since most of these foods are fruits and vegetables containing indigestible cellulose, hemicellulose, and lignin (roughage), one would expect that large amounts would irritate some people's digestive tracts while leaving others unscathed. In a humoral system it makes sense to call the former colder than normal, and to expect that their lists of cold foods will be more extensive than those of warmer people. Malays say, however, that even a normal person cannot live for long periods on large quantities of cold foods only, because he will eventually become weak. Since neither animal proteins nor fats are cold, we can assume that an entirely cold diet may lack complete proteins, concentrated food energy, and fat-soluble vitamins. It would not be surprising if such a diet caused a lack of energy.

Hot foods, I was told, make one feel satiated and healthy. Since many of these are fatty (providing nine calories per gram compared with four per gram for carbohydrates), and contain animal proteins (with a full complement of essential amino acids) one might expect this effect. Some people, however, whose high blood has already unbalanced their systems toward the hot polarity, cannot eat large quantities of hot foods without suffering headaches, dizziness, and blurred vision. All these can be indicative of hypertension, a condition aggravated by ingestion of large quantities of sodium. Salted fish, a hot food, might well bring on these symptoms.[12]

When I was collecting foods to be analyzed chemically at the Institute for Medical Research in Kuala Lumpur, most of my informants assumed that a laboratory analysis would reveal the humoral qualities of the foods as well as their nutritive content. The institute staff considered this an amusing conceit, yet a study

[49]

in India has shown that laboratory tests may indeed offer insights into humoral systems. Ramanamurthy (1969) put four individuals on hot diets (according to Indian humoral conceptions) for ten days, and then on cold diets for the same length of time. Subjective feelings reported during the hot diet were burning eyes, burning urination, and a general feeling of warmth in the body. Analysis of urine and feces showed that subjects on the hot diet displayed higher urine acidity and sulfur excretion and lower retention of nitrogen, although analyses of the diets for sulfur and nitrogen did not show any significant differences.[13]

THE HUMORS AND ILLNESS

Illnesses are classified by the following criteria, all of which interpret empirical evidence in the light of humoral reasoning:

1. *External heat.* Some hot illnesses, such as fever and boils, make the patient feel hot to the touch.

2. *Internal heat.* Other hot ailments make the patient feel internally hot or experience burning sensations, such as sore throat and heartburn.

3. *Imitation of people's reactions to atmospheric temperatures.* Malaria, which is characterized by violent chills and shudders, is called cold fever (*demam sejuk*).

4. *Visible signs.* A bloody nose is an obvious sign that the hot element has become overheated and boiled over. Clotted phlegm indicates that the cold element has become still colder.

5. *Deficiency or excess of one of the body humors, deduced from internal evidence.* Anemia is cold since its sufferers are lacking in blood, the hot humor. Vertigo and hypertension are hot since an excess of blood is presumed to have gone to the head, overheating it.

6. *Pulse reading.* A fast pulse denotes heat, since its speed is owing to the rate at which the blood travels through the veins. A

slow pulse is a sign that inner cold has thickened the blood, making it sluggish.

7. *Behavioral considerations.* Some forms of madness, characterized by violent behavior, are thought to occur when the head becomes overheated. Angry behavior, whether indulged in by the mad or the sane, is called *panas hati* (hot-livered, or hot-hearted). A person quick to anger has a hot liver (the seat of emotions) as well as a hot head.

8. *Response to treatments.* If illnesses respond to treatments classified as hot or cold, this shows that these illnesses have the opposite humoral quality. Asthma is cold since it responds to heat therapies such as steam inhalation; heatstroke, which responds to cold water applied internally and externally, is thereby hot.

9. *In reference to other humoral criteria.* Since rheumatism is most often found in old people (humorally colder than younger adults) it is classified as cold.

The Malay humoral system thus provides logical and empirically observable criteria for the classification of many disease states.[14]

Of Time and the Weather

Illnesses can be attributed to humoral variations related to changes of time and weather. A rise in the prevalence of upper respiratory and gastrointestinal diseases is noted when the seasons change and there is a significant rise or fall in the mean temperature. Malays say this happens because some people's bodies do not adjust quickly, leaving their inner temperature out of harmony with the outside world. Changes of season are, as well, interstitial times, neither exactly one thing nor another. People are thought to be particularly vulnerable during such times.

Dangerously ambiguous times also occur daily, and cautious

[51]

people guard against sudden changes in body temperature by not bathing at dawn, when night is changing into morning; at noon, when it is no longer morning, but not yet afternoon; and at dusk, when day is giving way to night. These are thought to be the hours when spirit activity is at its height and, since spirits success-fully attack only those whose vitality has been lowered, or whose vital life force (*semangat*) has been startled, subjecting one's body to the shock of cold well water would be imprudent. Similarly, people do not bathe immediately upon returning home after working in the hot sun, but wait until their bodies have cooled.[15]

Ambiguous weather can be potentially dangerous to health. Rain is associated with cold, sunshine with heat. So, when a sunshower occurs, the regularity and harmony of nature have been disturbed and may intensify disharmony within the human body. While healthy adults may not suffer ill effects from *hujan panas* (literally hot rain, the Malay term for sunshower), mothers fear the unnatural heat may cause fever in a sickly child.

The pattern of marked and unmarked features should now be clear. Interstitial, ambiguous times, seasons and weather condi-tions (marked features) are not dangerous per se, but only to people who are themselves in marked categories. People who become ill when the seasons change are those whose bodies are not in humoral balance; those who work in the hot sun find their humoral balance temporarily skewed from the unmarked norm to the hot polarity; healthy adults have little to fear from sun-showers, but sickly children, who are doubly marked—by age and ill health—cannot afford to be exposed to a marked feature from the domain of weather.

Humoral Treatments

Many conditions are thought to respond, negatively or posi-tively, to food. The types of food that should be avoided are common knowledge, reinforced or amended by consultation with

[52]

indigenous specialists. For a hot fever, it is wise to omit very hot food which will drive the fever still higher, and very cold food which would make the body ache. For a cold sickness, including many gastrointestinal conditions, people advise limiting the diet to rice, fish, and fish soup.

Some medical treatments can be classified on the basis of external criteria, such as the thermal temperature they employ therapeutically. Others are classified by the conditions that they treat, or by association with foods. Asthma, a cold condition, is treated by applying heat in as many ways as possible. A sufferer is encouraged to lie near a fire, drink coffee (both thermally and humorally hot), eat hot foods, and take hot medicines. One such medicine employs water buffalo meat, a hot food made still hotter by exposing it to a swarm of *kerengga* (*Oecophylla smaragdina*), red ants whose painful bite leaves a raised inflammation. As they walk over the meat and eat bits of it, they leave behind small amounts of urine and saliva that give the meat a strong taste. To insure that it loses none of its heat, the meat is cooked over direct heat instead of boiling it in water, an intrinsically cold element. The hot taste of the hot meat, combined with the memory of the *kerengga*'s hot bite, make this a potent remedy to balance the cold of asthma.

A fever may be eased by applying a cooling poultice of soursop leaves (*Annona muricata*). Many people place sticking plasters treated with menthol on their foreheads for headache and fever (both hot conditions). Bathing with water into which lime juice has been squeezed is a common treatment for headache and dizziness, thought to be symptomatic of heat concentration in the head. All these treatments actually do provide a feeling of coolness.

Other medicines are cold because they taste kelat (a criterion also used for foods), or by means of other associations. A father treated his baby's weeping eczema (hot) with gratings of soft stones from the cold river bed. A man with a gaping wound in his leg bathed it in sea water, since the heat of the salty water would

[53]

dry up the blood and encourage healing.[16] Friends reasoned that aspirins are cold because they reduce a hot fever. They can even be used as an antidote for medicine that has proven too hot. My assistant took an antihistamine for a runny nose, and then later asked for aspirin, saying the antihistamine had been so hot it had not only dried up his nose but his mouth and throat as well.

One of the treatments believed to be most effective for hot conditions was only part of local legend until I arrived. One day, after treating a neighbor's child for a spirit-induced illness, a bomoh came to my house to ask for an aspirin to ease his (naturally-caused) headache. During his visit, he noticed a still life setup that my husband was painting. His eye was caught by a stone egg, which looked like a real hen's egg. He had heard many times of stone eggs, which people of ancient times were supposed to have found in the hills, but he had never seen one. He offered to teach me some of his art in return for the egg. Before I left Malaysia I supplied many of the bomoh with stone eggs from China and Italy. I was told that they could be used not only for very high fevers but also for poisoning and lockjaw, both extremely hot conditions. Some bomoh dipped the eggs in water to make the water "colder." Others grated infinitesimal bits of the eggs, mixed them with cold grated roots, and added the mixture to water. The treated water was used to wash the patient's head, where the heat was most concentrated. Since it was new to their armamentarium, the bomoh experimented a great deal to see what conditions might be helped by a stone egg.

Although Malay medicines can be classified as hot or cold, none is as hot as some medicines dispensed at the hospital (but not all; e.g., aspirin is cold), the hottest of which is a shot of penicillin. The idea that many hospital drugs are hotter than indigenous varieties is used to explain why they are quicker and more effective. Thus, one must take special precautions when being treated with hospital drugs to avoid foods that are also extremely hot. Within days of my arrival I was told to avoid eating cassava root and durian when taking hospital-type drugs, lest I suffer the consequences of overheating: headache, dizziness, nausea, and blurred vision.

With some illnesses, the consequences of taking hospital drugs are believed to be much more serious. Measles cannot be treated with hospital medicine because the heat of the drugs will cause the disease to turn inward on the patient and make him very ill.[17] Even the village schoolteachers felt it was better to have a bomoh treat their children's measles with spells and cold remedies than to rely on doctors. When the rash appears on the skin, it signals the exit of heat from the patient's body.[18]

Buah and *barah*, two stomach conditions thought of as internal abcesses or tumors, cannot be treated with hot hospital drugs, since the combined heat of the disease and medication can cause death. Very high fevers can become more dangerous if treated with hot medicine. One young man was considered to have gone mad as a result of this intense heat, which had reached his brain and caused him to become *panas* (angry and violent as well as humorally and thermally hot). He was taken to a bomoh, who gave him cold medicine and recited cooling incantations. This treatment calmed him down (caused him to become less panas), so that he was no longer violent, but neither was he entirely normal in his behavior. People said his brain was permanently burned out.

Not all humoral treatments simply provide the patient with the opposite of the humoral quality of his illness. Sometimes, when the heat of the condition is not too strong, it is advisable to give hot medicines, following a homeopathic theory. Frequently medicines are mixed, providing hot and cold substances in one dose to make the mixture the right "temperature" for the illness. Some bomoh say it is important to match the qualities of illness and medicine, and easily assign humoral values to all components of each concoction. Others are less interested in a medicine's humoral quality than in whether or not it works. The latter admit,

[55]

with no loss of confidence in their healing powers, that the cause and cure of many ailments are a mystery. They may use a humoral idiom opportunistically (i.e., this medicine is probably cold because it brought down a fever), but they are essentially clinicians rather than theoreticians.[19]

EXTENSIONS OF THE MALAY HUMORAL SYSTEM

Malay humoral thought reaches far beyond the everyday concerns of diet, sickness, and treatment. Land, water, and metals are classified humorally. Sandy soil, found near the salty sea, is "hottest"; rich, muddy soil is "colder"; clay is "coldest." Among metals, gold and copper are hottest, followed by iron, silver, and tungsten; tin is coldest. Inland regions are said to be colder than areas near the shore, because of the cold air which people claim can be felt rising from the tin deposits underground, and the lack of warming properties the salt air imparts to breezes blowing over the ocean. Ocean water, since it is salty, is the hottest naturally occurring water, followed by river and well water. Rainwater is colder, except for sunshowers, which are unnaturally hot. Dew is coldest: staying out in the dew can lead to cold fevers.

People in inland regions are known to suffer more often from "cold fevers" (malaria) than those on the seaside. Malaria is now found primarily in edge areas near the jungle. In my parish, the only cases were in the hamlet closest to the jungle and furthest from the sea. The most important vector, *Anopheles maculatus*, is a night-feeder, shy of human habitation, whose feeding peaks about midnight (Sandosham 1959:144). Those who stay out when dew is on the ground, especially in inland regions, may well fall victim to its bite.

Spirits, Divination, and Exorcism

Humoral concerns permeate Malay theory regarding the nature of spirits, their influence on human well-being, and methods

[56]

of divination and treatment. *Hantu* most often afflict their human siblings by blowing their superheated breath on human backs, upsetting the victim's humoral balance and bringing on disease.

This view of supernaturally-caused illness is congruent both with the medieval Arabian view, which characterized fever as "an exhalation of Hell" (Browne 1921) and with aboriginal Malay exorcisms: "Be cold what was hot, be cold and cool" (Skeat and Blagden 1906:I, 695), and "Let go the demons and the devils that dwell within this flesh and sinews and let the hot grow cold" (Skeat and Blagden 1906, II:296). One of the meanings of panas is "unholy," particularly in reference to black magic (*ilmu panas*). Treatment for supernaturally induced illness involves restoring the natural balance of the elements by removing excess fire and air and increasing earth and water, but it does not involve dietary changes.

Before proceeding with the treatment, it is sometimes necessary to divine both cause and prognosis. This can be done by several methods, two of which are basically humoral. The first employs rice popped by dry heat. In the course of the healing ceremony, the shaman places handfuls of the popped rice on a pillow and counts out the grains in pairs, two each for earth, air, fire, and water. If the count ends on earth, it might point to a cold illness, or one caused by the spirits of the earth, or a particularly tenacious ailment. If it falls on fire, it might signify that the patient has incurred someone's hot wrath, whether human or genie, or it might simply mean that the condition was hot. The shaman usually knows a good deal about the patient and the circumstances surrounding his difficulties before he begins, and the many possible meanings for each category give him considerable leeway in diagnosis and prognosis.

Popped rice is also used to attract spirits to the seance, since the dry heat makes it humorally congruent with the hantu. It is used in conjunction with incense—heat and air whose smell is pleasing to the spirits. However, plain rice, the fruit of the irrigated earth, repels hantu.

[57]

Another method of divination is reading the flame of a bees-wax candle. No other type of candle can be substituted. The bee partakes of the hantu's unholy heat (as does honey, used only medicinally). Found in the jungle, beyond human control (at least on the east coast of Malaysia), and commanding a remarkably hot sting, bees are called the friends of the hantu.

The bomoh has several methods of increasing the cold and wet elements of the patient's body. Spells are recited with the patient's back to the healer. At strategic times during the recitation the bomoh blows on his patient's back. His breath, cooled by the incantation, counteracts the hot breath of the hantu. Bomoh frequently prescribe that the patient drink and bathe in magically treated water and lime juice, already cold and wet by their nature and made colder still by the bomoh's breath. Another powerful balancer is the rice paste used in many magical ceremonies. Made of rice—the quintessential fruit of the earth—which has been ground and mixed with water, the cold and wet properties of this paste are used to balance the excess fire and air of the hantu.

But the victim of a spirit attack becomes ill not only because the normal harmony within his body has been disrupted but also because things are out of place in the universe. Spirits should remain within their own domain and not encroach upon the world of the spirit made flesh. Besides restoring the balance of elements within the patient's body, the bomoh must exorcise the afflicting spirit and restore order in the universe. The bomoh's exorcism ends by exhorting the spirits to return to their place so that peace and health can once again reign in the universe and within Man, the universe in microcosm.

Sakit Berangin—The Sickness of Frustration

Many of the illnesses treated by shamans, while conforming to a humoral model, are believed to be caused neither by spirits nor by the types of impersonal systemic causes previously discussed.

These illnesses, called *sakit berangin* (wind sickness) are not caused by the wind that blows through the trees or by a magical wind sent by human or nonhuman enemies. Within the context of the shamanistic curing ceremony (Main Peteri), this is the wind that blows through the heart, an airy component of the four elements. *Angin* (wind or air) in this context is similar to temperament in medieval Europe. People are composed of earth, air, fire, and water, but all the elements are not necessarily present in equal amounts. Those with more fire are quicker to anger than those with a preponderance of earth or water. People with an over-abundance of air are more susceptible to sakit berangin.

We all possess angin—inherited characters, talents, and de-sires—but some have more, or stronger, angin. If such people can express their angin, they will lead untroubled lives and, in fact, may be among the community's most respected people by virtue of their strong and gifted characters. If they cannot ex-press themselves adequately, their angin gets shut up within them and may cause illness. A midwife or bomoh who is not popular can suffer from sakit berangin, as can a person who longs without success to act in the Malay opera, or even a masseur who does not have a steady call on his services. The most prevalent type, *Angin Dewa Muda* (Young Demigod), results when the desire to be attractive, pampered, and admired is frustrated. According to bomoh, many people have inherited this angin, but few can satisfy it fully. Symptoms of sakit berangin are similar to those in our own category of psychosomatic disorders: backaches, head-aches, digestive problems, dizziness, asthma, depression, and general malaise.

Malays believe that when angin builds up within the body, it destroys the balance of the four elements of which the world is made. The treatment of choice for sakit berangin is to put the patient in trance, allowing him to behave in ways that might ordinarily evoke public censure. Patients in trance laugh and cry, dance in the manner of the Malay opera (if that is their angin),

[59]

attempt to contact a spirit (if they have the unsatisfied angin of a bomoh), or flirt with the shaman (Laderman 1980). Acting out one's desires in an approved setting allows excess angin to escape from the body so that balance, and with it, health, can be restored. Because the etiologies of sakit berangin and spirit-induced illnesses are understood as not proceeding directly from the body, there are no accompanying food beliefs, avoidances, or proscriptions.

Markedness of Person, Role, and Language

Excessive heat as a metaphor for baleful influences extends beyond concerns for individual health to the health of the body politic. The successful rule of a Malay sultan is harmonious—the heat of war will not destroy the nation, the heat of anger will not cause internal dissension, and the heat of nature will not destroy the crops. Historically, the Malay ruler was considered to be as intimately connected to the unseen world and its control, on a national level, as the bomoh on an individual level.[20] State shamans were of royal descent, frequently brothers of the ruling sultan. The ruler himself kept familiar spirits. On important occasions within the last century sultans have officiated as shamans in seances of national importance (Winstedt 1951:9–11; Endicott 1970:94). The name and authority of the sultan is still invoked by villagers (without his permission) when confronted by a spirit whose power cannot be challenged by any lesser personage. The hamlet in which I lived was nicknamed Feverville (*Kampung Demam*) because of the high incidence of fevers. A bomoh divined that they were due to one of the Great Spirits who lived in a large tree in the middle of the hamlet. The only way to get rid of these fevers was to cut down the tree, thus depriving the *Hantu Raya* of his home. This, however, was very dangerous since the hantu was bound to resent their actions and take revenge. The solution was to counterfeit a letter from the sultan of Trengganu

[60]

ordering the villagers to cut down the tree and, in effect, giving the spirit his eviction notice. This letter, along with another, signed by the village headman, was placed in the crotch of the tree. The second letter explained that none of this was the fault of the people; they were only following orders.

The power of the Malay ruler to keep or restore peace and harmony within his kingdom rests, metaphorically, in his ability to provide the coolness that balances the destructive heat threatening the body politic. Within his own person, the successful sultan embodies this coolness, made explicit by such expressions as *Perentah-nya sejuk,* usually translated as "His reign was full of benign influences," but literally meaning "His reign was cold" (Zainal-Abidin 1947:43).

The ruler, the bomoh, and the ordinary man correspond to descending orders of markedness, both in their control over the forces of "heat" and in the language associated with them. Since the ruler embodies cooling balance and control, and is in every respect an uncommon person, the language used to him, by him, and in reference to him, is always the marked form. Ordinary people eat (*makan*), sleep (*tidur*), and die (*mati*). The ruler does none of these: he never eats, he regales himself (*bersantap*); disdaining sleep, he reposes (*beradu*); he does not die, he is wafted aloft (*mangkat*). Royal words are never used by commoners to refer to themselves. Indeed, in earlier times use of the royal personal pronoun by a commoner was a criminal offense (Wilkinson 1959:I, 132).

The bomoh is marked in his role rather than in his person. When not acting in his professional capacity, his speech is the ordinary language of everyday village life. In his role as master of spirits who, by virtue of his cooling remedies, can nullify destructive heat, he uses those marked forms that identify his language as ritual speech. He does not recite (*baca*) his spells, he incants them (*bangkit*); his words do not call (*panggil*) spirits, they summon (*aboh*). Just as the language of royalty is never employed toward

[61]

common people, so, too, the language of ritual is reserved only for encounters with the spirits.

The common man is marked neither in his person nor in his role, but can enter into a marked state with his prayers. The language of Malay prayer is not marked in the same manner as royal or ritual languages, which build their differences from the ordinary upon a base of everyday Malay. Prayer is offered in Arabic, the holy language of Islam, whose words are learned by rote. Village Malays understand their prayers in a general way, but cannot ordinarily tell you what any particular word means. Recitation of the "blessed cooling prayer" (Zainal-Abidin 1947: 43) takes the ordinary man out of the confines of profane existence and places him in the realm of the sacred. For the moment, he shares the cool polarity with the bomoh and the sultan and can be a force for universal harmony by balancing spiritual heat.

THE CONCEPT OF *BISA*

Less pervasive than the Malay humoral system, but even more important within its narrow range, is the concept of *bisa*. Like the humoral system, it is strengthened by observable phenomena that, by their force, carry along the belief system as a whole.

Wilkinson's (1959:I, 145) definition of bisa is "blood-poison, anything that gives a septic wound, venomous. Of the stings of hornets, scorpions and centipedes; the bites of snakes; the poison used on darts; the septic nature of bites of tigers and crocodiles; and of wounds from krises of laminated steel." This definition leaves out the core meaning of the term and neglects its most common usage.

Malays refer to magical power, whether used for good or evil, as bisa. The words of the bomoh, neutral when he is not speaking in his professional capacity, become bisa when he recites an incantation. The words of the sultan are always bisa to his subjects. Bisa connotes power. No judgment is implied concerning the nature of this power: the bomoh's bisa words are usually used for their curative power, although he may also use them to harm, and the ruler's bisa speech is for the well-being of the nation, although it may prove painful to some of his subjects. The word is used in spells for the expulsion of sickness to refer to inimical influences of any kind.

The most frequent use of the word is in connection with foods and food avoidances. This is not part of the humoral system, although it has been confused with it (Skeat 1972:343; Wilson 1971:96). Foods that are bisa and foods that are humorally "cold" are avoided simultaneously during certain disease states and life crises, particularly postcircumcision and postpartum. Dietary proscriptions for boys who have just gone through the rite of puberty are the same as those for women after parturition. These restrictions link the circumstances under which the sexes attain social maturity: for a male it is the rite of circumcision, which usually occurs during early adolescence; for a female it is neither circumcision (which occurs during infancy) nor menarche which is marked by observance among Malays; it is childbirth that turns a girl into a woman.

Food restrictions of all kinds are called *pantang* in Malay, a word frequently translated as *taboo* (see, e.g., Colson 1971 on this subject). Taboo, however, usually connotes something that is forbidden because of supernatural strictures and entails an extra-natural penalty, or at least a social one. Pantang might better be called guideposts for behavior, which leave the possibility for cautious experimentation open. Malay food pantang have no jural or moral force; those who do not observe them will not call down the wrath of God, the vengeance of spirits, or punishment from human sources. The dangers are natural and by no means invariable. A new mother who eats food considered bisa and experiences no harmful consequences may even be complimented on her "cast-iron" stomach; and a woman who experiences postpartum hemorrhage or stomachache after eating bisa

[63]

food is not considered a sinner, merely a bit of a fool.[21]

Malays do not think of bisa foods as toxic or poisonous but rather as intensifiers of disharmonies already present within the body. Bisa foods have the power to aggravate a preexistent problem. Foods are not bisa per se, but only in context and, even then, some people have constitutions so strong that they can eat them safely.

Social scientists have treated the concept of bisa as a laundry list devoid of structure (Wilson 1970, 1971), or as symbolism "succinctly expressive of the patient's dilemma as a social being. The symbolism is that of impure food. The bomoh usually extends the symbolism of the performance by prescribing a detailed diet for the patient" (Provencher 1971:188–189). Wilson (1970:338) allies herself with medical orthodoxy by asserting that these beliefs are detrimental to health because she assumes that the long list of proscribed foods interferes with nutritional health. Millis (1958:141), a Malaysian nutritionist, is specifically concerned about postpartum protein intake, because mollusks, crustaceans, and many varieties of fish are considered bisa during the forty days following childbirth. The consequences of acting on these beliefs have never been examined, but rural people believe that avoiding bisa foods has a beneficial effect on health. Knowledge of which foods are bisa is fairly standardized. People act upon it during illnesses and in other vulnerable conditions. Individuals who experience adverse reactions when they eat foods that are not commonly thought to be bisa say that for them these foods also belong to this category.

Two beliefs about bisa accord well with what we know about allergies. First, allergic reactions occur only after the patient has been sensitized to a particular allergen, and may either be lifelong or transient. Malays believe that bisa foods have a relationship to preexistent disharmonies within an individual. He is usually aware of his condition but, in some cases, the illness may hide within the person's body unknown to him and emerge only when a bisa food is eaten.

[64]

Second, patients with allergic disorders have an inherited tendency to develop sensitivity to certain substances that are harmless to others. Similarly, although most people avoid certain foods on the standard bisa list only during periods of special vulnerability, some individuals avoid them at all times, usually because of digestive disturbances.

It would be a mistake, however, to assume that bisa and allergen are synonymous. Many of my Malay neighbors developed red, itchy welts after eating albacore or Spanish mackerel. For them, these fish were bisa. Their reaction may have been due to scombroid poisoning. The flesh of fish normally contains a chemical constituent called histadine, found in varying amounts in different species. When histadine is acted upon by bacteria it changes into saurine, a histamine-like substance which can cause an illness resembling severe allergy. Scombroid fishes, which include albacore and Spanish mackerel, are especially prone to become toxic when left to stand in the sun, or even room temperature in the tropics (Halstead 1959:112), but do not cause illness when fresh. With this in mind it becomes significant that native healers advise patients not to eat stale fish. Their dietary recommendations may be grounded in the reality, as well as the symbolism, of impure food.[22]

Other reasons for regarding foods as bisa appear to have symbolic content—for example, the prohibition against eating fruit (buah) when one has the disease called *sakit buah*. Since the name is the same, I was told, adding one to the other will exacerbate the condition. Sick people avoid watermelon and cucumbers since they grow close to the ground and must be manured. Malays believe the association with manure is unhealthy for vulnerable people. Similarly, chickens are considered bisa by some for young children because they eat feces and other dirty things and also, because village fowl regularly contract many illnesses, parents fear that eating even healthy specimens may, by extension, make their children sick.

In general, precautions about bisa foods come into play when a person has entered a condition that is an extreme example of a marked feature. For example, a person afflicted with a common skin disease such as scabies does not have to avoid bisa foods, but one with *badan*, a rare skin condition that looks like severe eczema, must eliminate these foods from his diet. Simple digestive problems do not ordinarily involve bisa restrictions, but *sakit buah* and *sakit barah*, two conditions considered by Malays to be life-threatening abcesses or tumors in the stomach, do call for these restrictions. Bleeding from minor wounds is a common occurrence and does not involve dietary changes; neither does menstruation. It is only the marked forms of genital bleeding that accompany important rites of passage—circumcision and child-birth—that involve both ritual and food avoidances according to humoral concepts as well as that of bisa.

Bisa Fish

The concept of bisa is clearest and most complete during postpartum and postcircumcision periods. Until the wound of circumcision is healed, a boy adheres to the same diet prescribed for the postparturient woman. They avoid sour fruits, cucumbers, and watermelon, humorally "cold" fruits and vegetables, fried foods, mollusks, crustaceans, and an extensive list of fish.[23] The midwife refers to these fish in particular when she cautions her patients about eating bisa. A number of reasons were given by informants for classifying a fish as bisa. The possession of any one of the following features is enough, but they become more compelling when several overlap.[24]

    I. Bisa fish have inconsistent features in comparison with normal "safe" (non-bisa) fish:
      A. Thick skin and thin scales (e.g., dolphin fish).
      B. Thin skin and thick scales (grunters).
      C. Scales larger than usual for their size (parrot fish, wrasse).

[66]

    D. They are spotted or speckled (threadfin).
  II. Bisa fish have threatening features:
    A. Venomous spines (catfish eel).
    B. Sharp but not venomous spines (climbing perch).
    C. Small, sharp bones that are hard to remove (wolf herring).
    D. Red (sometimes yellow) color, reminiscent of blood (red snapper).[25]
  III. Bisa fish have disturbing eating habits.
    A. They are bottom feeders (bream).
    B. They eat organisms poisonous to people, such as jellyfish and annelid worms (Spanish mackerel).
  IV. Bisa fish are associated with the "cold" humor (*lendir*).

Fish with particularly slimy skin, such as catfish (which are also bottom feeders), belong in this category. They may also belong in category II for reasons to be discussed.

All bisa fish are marked, that is, they have characteristics that distinguish them from unmarked "safe" fish.[26] The safe fish are the most common and most abundant species, easy to catch, inexpensive and available for sale on an almost daily basis.

The first three criteria for bisa fish in Category I fit nicely into Douglas's theory of the danger of anomalies (1966). When measured against safe fish, bisa fish are inconsistent. If skin is thick, scales should be thick as well, and vice versa—mixing features is anomalous and therefore dangerous. Rejecting the parrot fish and wrasse for the abnormal size of their scales implies a standard of normality, embodied by the unmarked species.

Criteria in Category II are primarily those of danger from piercing spines or bones. People who recently have undergone experiences believed to create wounds on or within their bodies, such as circumcision or childbirth, will avoid these associations.

The final criterion in Category II relates to the laws of magic (Frazer 1959:7). Like begets like, therefore, since red is the color of blood, eating red foods may, by homeopathic magic, cause postpartum hemorrhage, delay the healing of the wound of circumcision, and encourage the angry red of infection. Yellow is also associated with blood in Malay magic.

Homeopathic reasoning may hold true as well for the feeding habits of bisa fish: those that eat dirty or poisonous substances will themselves be dirty or poisonous.

Slimy (berlendir) fish are associated with the cold humor. Childbirth and circumcision involve loss of blood, the hot humor, from the genitals, making the patient humorally cold. Since the essence of humoral pathology is to restore balance within the body, cold foods are restricted in the diets of people in a cold state. Aside from its humoral coldness, fish slime is an irritant and source of infection to preexistent wounds (see Halstead 1959: 91–92 for corroboration of indigenous observation). Since the postpartum period is conceived of as a time for healing internal wounds, it is not surprising that a substance known to be antithetical to surface wounds would be avoided by women who have recently given birth (although ichthyologists assert that there is no connection between touching fish slime—a possibly dangerous procedure—and eating the flesh of such fish, which carries no peril).

Spotted or speckled fish are bisa, I was told, because of their ancestors' quarrelsome nature. As Malays explain, during the Great Flood certain fish continually fought among themselves. Noah punished them by striking them on their sides, leaving spots and speckles that can be seen on their descendants to this day.

Obviously, the categorization of bisa fish is symbolic, but avoidance seems also to have an extrasymbolic basis. For example, in my east coast parish the only fishes considered to have abnormally large scales are the wrasses and parrot fishes. Besides being symbolically ambiguous, the flesh of these fish spoils easily, causing choleralike symptoms in those who eat it (C. Lavett Smith 1978, personal communication). Also, eating spiny fish can be perilous, aside from the danger of handling them. Two of these fish, *ikan barat-barat* (*Ballisteodei*) and *ikan jebong* (*Abalistes stellaris*) are close kin of the puffer and porcupine fishes, known to carry tetra-ondontoxin, a powerful nerve poison that occasionally causes fatalities in Japan (Halstead 1959:113–115).

Avoiding bottom feeders during vulnerable periods appears to be based, in good measure, on empirical reality. Malaysia is within the belt of ciguatera-producing fish. Ciguatera is a type of poisoning produced by a large variety of tropical marine fishes that are mainly bottom feeders (Halstead 1967:II, 605). Ichthyologists believe that these fish become poisonous because of their feeding habits. Ciguatoxic fish, constituting more than one-sixth of those species considered bisa, tend to be large carnivores, at the apex of the food pyramid. Having eaten smaller fish, which have eaten still smaller fish, which have eaten the blue-green algae thought to carry ciguatera, these large fish concentrate the poison within their flesh and become more virulent than animals farther down on the food chain. In humans, the symptoms of ciguatera poisoning include extreme weakness, vomiting, diarrhea, and abdominal cramps. Mortality has been estimated at from 7 to 60 percent (Halstead 1959:116; Craig 1980:273), and those who recover may be debilitated for more than six months (C. Lavett Smith 1978: personal communication).

Two other bisa species (*ikan tiram* [*Clupea kangurta*], and *ikan pisang-pisang* [*Albula vulpes*]) may be implicated as a source of clupiotoxication, which causes symptoms similar to those of ciguatera (Halstead 1967:II, 619). Rays, another bisa fish, have been known to be ichthyosarcotoxic (Halstead 1967:II, xxx). The virulence of these poisons is not altered by cooking, salting or drying (Halstead 1967:II, 286, 619).

The list of safe fish is equally revealing. Compared with fifty-four bisa species, everyone agrees on the safety of six species, to which many add another thirteen. None of the fish on this list is scombroid or suspected of toxicity. None is a top carnivore, and all are rather small species, well out of the ciguatoxic category. The list of safe fish represents the most abundantly available varieties, including two that can be caught in any swampy area or padi field. In contrast, fish on the bisa list tend to be large, relatively rare, more difficult to catch, and expensive. One is unlikely to find most of them offered for sale in the village, whereas some variety of safe fish is usually available daily. Therefore, although the list of bisa fish is far longer than that of safe fish, it involves no nutritional sacrifice to do without them, even for extended periods.

Unmarked categories of foods (fresh fish and rice in the humoral system, safe fish in the bisa system) are those essential for life, while marked categories are supplementary, and thus easy to reduce or remove from the diet.

Malay beliefs in general and pantang, both behavioral and dietary, in particular, have built-in flexibility. Rather than being perceived as a sword of Damocles threatening to strike those who do not obey their admonitions, pantang are tested by some, ignored by others, and followed implicitly by the rest. The consequences of not following them are considered by no means invariable.

Negative cases, such as women in the puerperium who have eaten bisa fish without experiencing problems, do not affect belief in the validity of the system. Malays reason that some people are so strong, or lucky, that they can get away with dangerous actions. The epidemiology of scombroid, ciguatera, and other fish poisoning offers ideal support for these beliefs.

Scombroid poisoning does not invariably occur when a person eats scombroid fish, and does not affect every victim with equal severity; ciguatera, clupiotoxication, and other forms of ichthyosarcotoxication are not invariable after eating implicated species. The incidence and severity of these illnesses depend on the potential victim's state of health prior to ingestion, as well as the level of toxicity in the individual fish, and the amount eaten.

[70]

Although more than three hundred different species have been incriminated in ciguatera, its occurrence is unpredictable and therefore exceedingly difficult to control (Halstead 1959:117). An occasional health problem associated with specimens of a particular species can be enough to place the entire species, and possibly related species as well, in the bisa category. Within any species, only some individuals are toxic. Of two caught simultaneously in the same place, one could be eaten without any ill effects and the other could produce agonizing symptoms (Gordon 1977:223). The variable nature of these problems supports rather than vitiates Malay belief regarding sickness and health.

SYMBOLIC OR PRAGMATIC?

Is the concept of bisa a symbolic device for the avoidance of ambiguity and cognitive dissonance, or does it codify pragmatic action? Of the fifty-four species of bisa fish, one-third are implicated in toxic reactions. The food habit criterion for bisa is congruent with objective facts: Ciguatoxic fish are carnivorous bottom feeders. Thus, bisa may codify pragmatic action, particularly when one adds the species that are included because of visual or behavioral associations with toxic species, for this simplifies the decision-making process during periods of vulnerability. But what about the fish included solely because of symbolic reasons? Those that are dangerous to touch because of their venomous spines or irritating slime are not poisonous to eat. Fish that have "inconsistent" features or disturbing coloration are dangerous only because of their ambiguity or symbolic associations, and have not been implicated in poisoning.

All bisa fish have elements of symbolic danger, but some that combine the features of symbolic and real danger may be significant health problems, especially to individuals recently stressed. One might paraphrase Lévi-Strauss (1963b:89) by saying that all bisa fish are "bad to think" and some are "bad to eat" as well.

[71]

Analysis of either the pragmatic or symbolic nature of such a system is rather like examination of an elephant's hindquarters or its head: one does not arrive at a valid picture of the beast as a whole. The dynamic nature of the symbolic system provides a structure for individual variability of action reminiscent of the musical structure of a chaconne. Although the ground bass repeats endlessly throughout the piece (like the basic ideas of the humoral system), the upper voices weave variation after variation above it. The effect is that of rich order, rather than either chaos or stasis.

The Malay humoral system and the concept of bisa are joined in the Malay world view—a vision of the universe composed of the elements of earth, air, fire, and water in harmonious opposition. The world, the state, and Man, the universe in microcosm, function optimally as long as equilibrium is maintained. Problems occur when the balance of opposing elements is disturbed. Checks and balances are provided to retain or restore essential equilibrium. The concept of bisa complements the humoral system. Abstractly it is pure power with no moral implications. Concretely it is an intensifier that exacerbates existing disharmonies. The language and theory of these systems are consistently used throughout a number of domains.

The humoral system provides metaphors for reasoning and understanding. When the kingdom prospers it is because the ruler is cool. When patients respond to the bomoh's incantations it is because the heat of the spirits has been nullified by the bomoh's coolness. At the same time, direct sensory experience reinforces the system by mooring it in reality. This "proof" of the system's validity is most persuasive when it occurs in the context of illness, or in other situations perceived to be dangerous or life-threatening; and when effect follows closely after cause. The symbolic structure makes experiences meaningful, but without the input from empirical reality the edifice would crumble.

[72]

· 4 ·

Conception and Pregnancy

Menarche is not a ritual occasion in Merchang. No celebrations mark the day, no food restrictions are observed, and girls may perform their usual household tasks. It is neither a time for rejoicing nor a time for taboos, since it is not first menstruation but childbirth that constitutes the significant event that changes a girl into a woman. Menstruation begins when a girl becomes *pandai*, which usually means skilled or clever but in this case refers to the attainment of a developmental stage. She is now a candidate for marriage. Public opinion, her own growing dignity, and her increasing acceptance of the role she will soon play—that of the modest and diffident Malay wife—now prevent her from bathing naked with her brothers and playing rough and tumble games with the boys, as little girls do. Many girls begin to wear long skirts in early adolescence.

A scanty menstrual flow is considered unhealthy, and girls are encouraged to eat sweet things to increase the flow. Each month blood from the heart is thought to drip down into the uterus, where it collects. Since the amount is limited, a copious flow will shorten the menstrual period. This is important because a woman cannot pray during menses. She is put into a state of ritual impurity by the escape of fluids from her genitals. Semen can be washed away, but the menstrual flow is more or less continuous.

[73]

Some girls paint a spot of blood from their first period on each of three steps leading to their house in the hope that this will limit their periods to three days.

Men are not supposed to have sexual intercourse with their wives at this time because of religious proscriptions and the notion that it could damage their genitals. Yet, according to several informants, if the husband wishes intercourse, the wife will not refuse. Some men boast about the practice, and a few claim that it can restore vigor to a man with potency problems.[1]

Menstrual blood is considered dirty, unlike the blood of one's flesh. Because of its uncleanness and bad smell, it does not attract the dangerous attentions of the Earth Spirit (Jin Tanah) and his company, who like the sweet blood of parturition. Thus, no protective rituals are necessary during menstruation. The normal period is not considered a time of illness (unlike the American conception of my childhood: "being unwell"). Because it prevents the performance of daily prayer, however, it is called the curse of Eve. Menstruation originated when Eve ate the forbidden fruit which, because of its toxicity, turned into menstrual blood. Other bodily functions, including defecation and urination, were also created at the moment when the forbidden fruit was eaten. Adam, less greedy than Eve, did not eat all the fruit. A piece of it stuck in his throat and became the Adam's apple.

CONCEPTION

Unlike preliterate people who believe it takes a number of acts of intercourse to form and nourish a baby, Malays consider one act, performed at the proper time, sufficient. This belief is part of the Malay "hot/cold" system (see chap. 3). Conception can take place only when both parents' bodies are in a "cool" state, an event that occurs once each month but is not affected by the woman's menstrual period. It can only happen on "the day the seeds fall" (*hari jatuh benih*), which can occur on either the first, second, third, fourteenth, fifteenth, sixteenth, twenty-eighth, twenty-ninth, or thirtieth of each Islamic month. Since no one knows in advance which will be the fateful day, people who want to conceive have intercourse on all of these days. One may get a clue to the real hari jatuh benih for a particular month, since on that day sexual desire is said to be particularly urgent. One bidan (midwife) explained to me that this is not an infallible sign because desire may arise for other reasons.

The median age at marriage for women is fifteen, and for first pregnancy sixteen (see tables 1 and 2). By the age of sixteen, 74 percent of all women I interviewed were married, and 70 percent were pregnant or had already given birth. However, before conception takes place in the mother's womb, the father has been pregnant for forty days. Men clearly remember craving foods shortly before their wives began to exhibit this and other signs of pregnancy. The baby begins life not as a creation in the mother's belly, but in the father's brain. This theory is expressed in incantations (*jampi*) recited by bomoh to ease difficult births:[2]

> Gabriel guarded the seed of life for 40 days. Its name was Light of Faith (Nur Din). Then Gabriel put it into the father's brain for 40 days. Its name was Light of God (Nur Allah). It fell to his eyes, Gleaming Light (Nur Cahaya), fell to his chest, True Sultan of Happy Feelings, navel of the world, fell to the big toe, King Phallus is its name. Then you pray 40 times a day, 40 times a night. Then you stay within the father 40 days, *di wadi mani manikam* (elements of spermatic fluid). From *di* comes earth, from *wadi* comes water, from *mani* comes fire, from *manikam* comes air. Then you are thrust into the mother's womb.

This portion of a birth incantation is a clear metaphoric statement about the essential nature of male and female. Humanity is formed of earth and partakes of animal nature (*hawa nafsu*), but also possesses rationality (*akal*), which makes us higher than the angels.[3] Although both men and women have akal and hawa nafsu, developed states of self-control and rationality are masculine qualities, while bodily emotions and hungers are associated with women. Since the baby is formed in the father's brain, it receives akal from a highly developed source. When it goes to the father's eyes and is called Nur Cahaya, reference is made to a common affectionate term, *cahaya mata* (light of my eyes). Malay mystics and practitioners of Main Puteri, the east coast shamanistic healing ceremony, consider the eyes to be the baby's first human attribute. In the Main Puteri the eyes are personified as guardians of the body. As the baby arrives at the father's chest, the microcosmic center of the universe, it comes to the dwelling place of the *hati*, repository of the emotions.[4] After the baby has experienced the father's rationality and emotions, it descends to the penis and is thrust into the mother's womb, the dark matrix of our animal nature. There, according to the village midwives and most of the lay people I spoke to, the baby finds a resting place, like a seed planted in the nourishing earth. Already formed from the four elements of its father's semen, the same four elements of which the world is made, it develops in its mother's body until it emerges like a flower into the light.

Partial disagreement with this theory came from bomoh, who are acknowledged to have more learning than midwives, whose "inner knowledge" is usually limited to the rituals of pregnancy and childbirth. Bomoh claim that the baby is incomplete as it makes its way through the father's body, and awaits the addition of the mother's earth, air, fire, and water before it develops into a human being. A bomoh's wife confirmed her husband's statements by referring to her chickens. The hen lays an egg, she pointed out, without the help of a rooster, but it takes both of them together to bring life to the egg. If everything depended upon the male, and the female was just the source of nourishment, the hen, she felt, would not be able to lay even a sterile egg. Inside the egg must be the female's di wadi mani manikam.

CONTRACEPTION AND ABORTION

In 1975, according to the government midwife's records, thirty women had accepted the birth control pill out of a population of over 1,000 potential users. Some women on the pill were embarrassed about it and asked that the fact be kept secret from their neighbors. The primary reasons given for not using the pill were worries that it would cause headache, backache, dizziness, and excessive vaginal discharge, which would repel husbands. Fear was also expressed that the pills would not dissolve in the stomach and would accumulate until they had to be removed by surgery. Although the government midwife exhibited examples of IUDs and condoms at her antenatal clinic, neither appealed to her audience. The idea of a foreign body being placed more or less permanently within the uterus suggested an operation. Surgery terrifies Malays and is a component of their unease concerning treatment at the hospital. Condoms were rejected by the men because of their anesthetizing qualities, cost, and association with prostitutes. Withdrawal was not in favor because it reduces satisfaction and is thought to cause nervousness.

Although few couples used Western-approved contraceptive methods, many were interested in limiting or spacing their children, particularly after the fifth baby was born. One of the methods prescribed by village midwives is abstinence during the hari jatuh benih. Although these days may or may not correspond to fertile periods, the method would cause abstinence for at least nine days out of every month, and more if none of these days fell during the menstrual period.

Many women rely on spells to keep from conceiving:

> In the name of God, the loving and merciful.
> White phlegm (semen), phlegm like stone, I want to crush you.[5]
> I stop at the hill, the hill breaks into bits.
> I stop at the stone, the stone becomes an arrow.

[77]

I stop at the grass, the ground becomes bare.
Hey, liquid, I want you to be liquified.
If you do not become liquid you are disloyal to Allah.
Not by my power, but by the holy words
There is no God but Allah and Muhammad is his Apostle.

The images of barrenness and sterility, and the command to
liquify the embryonic blood, are striking. Success in magic is said
to be contingent on faith for its efficacy, but this does not prevent
the woman who taught me this spell from rising immediately
after intercourse to massage her abdomen downward while
jumping, in an effort to expel the sperm. Perfect faith, while
important, cannot assure success. In the Malay cosmic scheme,
effect does not always follow after cause. Faith increases the odds,
but it never hurts to help it along by whatever method one can.

Operating on the theory that coolness is necessary for conception, some women drink "hot" medicines for their supposed
contraceptive qualities and some use them as an abortifacient.
The fetus is considered to be a clot of blood in the early stages,
and hot medicine is thought to liquify the blood, and to make the
womb uncongenial for the child.[6]

A mechanical method of contraception involves turning the
uterus shortly after a woman has given birth. Thus, in the future,
sperm would not have a straight path to their destination. One old
bomoh specialized in this procedure. He learned the method
while visiting the neighboring state of Pahang, and had practiced
it with a limited clientele for about four years. For three successive
days during the week after childbirth, while the uterus is still large
and palpable, the bomoh comes in the morning to massage and
slowly turn the uterus. After reciting a jampi and ritually indicating the four cardinal directions on the woman's abdomen, he
massages the uterus for about thirty minutes. At the end of each
session the uterus is visibly displaced, and after three days of
treatment, it seems to be 45 degrees from its normal position,
with the fundus pointing toward the right and the cervix to the

[78]

left. The procedure is painless. The bomoh claims that it can be used also on women who have not recently given birth, but is then considerably more uncertain and difficult because the uterus is small and has receded into the body cavity. The practitioner and his patients claimed that turning the uterus resulted in sterility for four years or more. I did not find any dissatisfied customers, but only a few women had had this treatment. Four American gynecologists to whom I described this operation told me that they doubted that turning the uterus would be effective as a method of contraception because the uterus is mobile following delivery, and no matter how much it is moved it probably would not stay where it was placed.

Rosemary Firth (1966:13) wrote that "abortion is regarded with horror by good Moslems." This implies that abortion at all stages of pregnancy is considered equally reprehensible, however, many people in Merchang believe that during the first two months, when the fetus is only coagulated blood with no human characteristics, abortion is not a sin. The appearance of the conceptus, when spontaneous or induced abortion occurs at this early stage of pregnancy, reinforces this belief. One popular method of inducing abortion is ingestion of "hot" and "sharp" substances. The combination of young pineapple, yeast, and black pepper is supposed to be an effective abortifacient (see Ngin 1975:83 for its use among Malaysian Chinese, and Burkill 1966:153 for its use in India). Pineapple, especially when unripe, is sharp because of the astringency of its juice, black pepper, like all spices, is hot, and yeast is one of the hottest foods available. It is used to turn cassava root into tapai, whose alcoholic content warms the eater. As fermentation proceeds, the yeast bubbles like slowly boiling water, graphically illustrating its heat. Symbolically, this combination of hot and sharp should produce an effective abortifacient. Experience, in this case, supports belief. Unripe pineapple contains a poisonous substance which acts as a violent purge. Taken in large quantities with yeast on an empty stomach, it can cause strong uterine contractions (Burkill 1966:152–153). Such empirical verification of symbolic truth is important for the maintenance of the symbolic system.

Another home remedy, the juice of *akar celaka* (accursed root, *Plumbago indica*) is drunk by women in Merchang in their attempts at early abortion.[7] Botanists, noting its widespread use throughout Asia, have termed Plumbago a strong and possibly dangerous abortifacient (Burkill 1966:1805–1807; Perry 1980: 317). Although it is not used as an "abortion stick" in Merchang, elsewhere the root is placed in the *os uteri*, where it stimulates prostaglandin production, which can cause placental separation (Gimlette and Thomson 1971:42).

These measures are thought to work only if the fetus is not *sayang* (comfortable, firmly fixed). Most Merchang women whose attempts at abortion fail must reconcile themselves to their pregnancies, since none of the local midwives can offer them any other solution. A truly desperate woman may find help farther afield. For example, a woman who had been a junior wife was divorced by three talak given at once. In this form of divorce, a couple may not remarry unless the wife has first married and been divorced by another man. Nevertheless, the woman continued to consort with her former husband surreptitiously (or so she imagined, but it was common knowledge among her neighbors). She became pregnant, to her dismay. An illegitimate child would have been a disgrace to her children, some of whom were marriageable girls. She herself, and her former husband, could have been arrested for khalwat. A quick remarriage was out of the question for the guilty couple, so this woman tried the pineapple cure, which had worked for her a year earlier but now failed. She went to a private clinic in Kuala Trengganu to ask for a shot to bring on her menstrual period, but this too was unsuccessful. She was afraid to consult a practitioner at the General Hospital because abortion is illegal in Malaysia. When all efforts to rid herself of this unwanted pregnancy had failed, the couple hired an interim husband to marry and quickly divorce the woman. Three months after the divorce the original couple could remarry, ensuring the baby's legitimacy at birth.

During the iddah period, after her cinabuta marriage, the woman heard of a famous female bomoh, living more than twenty-five miles from Merchang, who, people said, could induce abortion. The bomoh started the treatment by massaging the woman's legs, lower back and abdomen. She recited a jampi, calling on Allah, Mohammad, Ali, and Abu Bakar to dissolve the fetus, certainly a sign that she did not feel her actions constituted a sin. She gave her patient the following material to boil and drink, a potful a day for three days:

> Akar 'pat punga (unidentified)
> Akar tunjung bumi (unidentified)
> Akar kacip Fatimah (*Labisia pothoina*)
> Akar teja jantan (probably a variety of cinnamon)
> Akar tapak leman (*Elephantopus scaber*)
> Akar siak (probably *Dianella ensifolia*)
> Akar pagar anak (*Semos chinepsis*)
> Bunga pala (*Myristica fragrans*—mace)
> Pucok baik (unidentified)
> Naga setus (*Vetiveria zizanoides*)

The ingredients in this mixture are extremely "hot." None is recorded as an abortifacient in the literature (Burkill 1966; Burkill and Haniff 1930; Gimlette and Burkill 1930; Gimlette and Thomson 1971), but most are used postpartum, when hot medicines are also prescribed.

When three days had passed, the woman returned as instructed for another deep massage. The bomoh felt her belly and assured her that she would abort within the week. The next day she told her friends that her troubles were over. There was now no need to remarry her former husband, and no evidence of their illicit lovemaking to embarrass them.[8]

Women who are anxious to carry their babies to term avoid

[81]

akar kayu and other hot medicines, such as penicillin. Cautious women, during the early months of pregnancy, may also be wary about eating much durian, because of its heating qualities, and jackfruit, because it is known to cause digestive problems. Fevers, which cause heat to descend from the naturally warm head to the womb, may also induce abortion. In an effort to avert this possibility, feverish women place cooling medicines on their heads. If a woman is beaten, or falls, striking her spine, a miscarriage might ensue. Such a blow, say the village midwives, could dislodge the placenta from its moorings to the backbone.

These dangers to the safety of the fetus carry an increased risk rather than a certainty of dire consequences. If the baby is *sayang*, it will probably survive. However, it is always prudent to call a bomoh to recite protective *jampi*, and to visit the bidan to make sure the baby is lying comfortably within the womb. None of the many herbal remedies of the traditional Malay pharmacopoeia is a specific against spontaneous abortion; many are employed after the event, to control bleeding.

When I bled profusely in the middle of my menstrual cycle, a bidan, diagnosing it as miscarriage, gave me a cold potion to drink composed of:

> Akar belalang puak (*Pittosporum ferrugineum*)
> Akar kacang sekucok (*Crotolaria striata*)
> Kemian (*Styrax benzoin*)

She then bruised the leaves of the first two ingredients and added them, together with pulverized shallots and black cumin seeds, to a pail of water which she directed me to pour over my head to decrease the dizziness which accompanied the bleeding. Within an hour after this treatment the bleeding tapered off and stopped, and the dizziness disappeared. Whether this was due to coincidence, suggestion, or the medicine is open to dispute.

A fetus aborted before the fifth month is not buried formally.

Conception and Pregnancy

Unable to move and still sharing its mother's soul, it is not yet an individual human being. After the fifth month, a fetus is given an Islamic burial.

The average interval between births in Merchang is two to three years (see table 5). This cannot be attributed to extensive

TABLE 5
BIRTH INTERVALS

Years between births*	%
One	13
Two	31.5
Three	35
Four	10
Five	5
Six	1.5
Seven	3
	99.0 N = 281

*Allowance has been made for fetal wastage and stillbirths. Fetal wastage reported was 26 out of a total of 566 live births. This is considerably lower than fetal wastage reported in the West, where a common rule of thumb is that 100 pregnancies produce roughly 88 live births, 10 miscarriages, and 2 stillbirths (Potter 1963:158), and probably reflects unreported and/or unrecognized early abortions.

induced abortions or high levels of spontaneous abortion. Studies have shown that more than half the women having regular intercourse without the intervention of contraception can expect to conceive within three months (Potter and Parker 1964:103). Nursing on demand can lengthen the anovulatory period considerably. The average duration of amenorrhea in nursing mothers in Central Java, for example, is 18.7 months (Mosely 1977:102). Allowing nine months for gestation, this would put the average

[83]

birth interval for such a population at about two and a half years as a natural function of lactational amenorrhea plus conceptive delay. Almost without exception, Merchang women nurse their babies for extended periods (see tables 6 and 7), and the average interval between births is exactly what might be expected under the circumstances.

TABLE 6

BREASTFEEDING AND BOTTLEFEEDING

N = 123

Breast only	Mixed	Bottle only**
75% (92)	22% (27)*	3% (4)*

*Twelve percent (15) used bottles for convenience, to be able to work or otherwise leave the house occasionally. Ten percent (12) used bottles because they felt their own milk supply was insufficient.
**Two percent (3) stopped nursing because they "had no milk." One percent (1) stopped because "it made her baby vomit."

TABLE 7

AGE AT WEANING FROM BREASTFEEDING*

N = 106	%	No.
1 year	6	6
between 1 year—1½ years	10	11
1½ years	16	17
between 1½—2	9	10
2 years	47	50
more than 2 years	11	12
	99%	

*Those few who stopped within days or weeks after delivery are not included.

Conception and Pregnancy

GESTATION

After intercourse on a "day the seeds fall," the opening of the womb closes, glued shut by a mixture of seeds and reproductive fluids which will keep the menstrual blood from escaping each month during pregnancy, and any further semen from entering during that time. At first the baby is only a mixture of liquids, but by the end of a month it has become a lump of blood. This belief, stemming from observations of early abortion and developing chicken eggs (one woman pointed out the blood spot in a fertilized egg, remarking that it was exactly like a human fetus in the first month), is reinforced by such Koranic statements as:

> Read in the name of the Lord who created,
> Who created man of blood coagulated.
> [(Sura 96:1–5)]

During the first two months the midwife cannot feel the embryo in the mother's womb. Pregnancy is suspected when a woman's breasts ache and her face turns pale, she craves sour foods, and her periods cease. Nausea and tiredness, while not indicative in themselves, give added proof of the woman's condition.

The sex of the baby is determined at the time of its conception in its father's brain, but its sex can be changed through the power of God. A family with children of only one sex is incomplete. To get a baby of the opposite sex, the parents may make a vow to hold a communal feast (*kenduri*) if God grants their request. Such vows are believed to carry severe consequences for those who break them: the child may be sickly all its life, or hemorrhage badly when circumcised.

The fetus is not the sole occupant of the womb. Its sibling, the placenta, develops during the second month.[9] At first they almost touch, but as the baby grows he moves away from his placental brother. The umbilical cord develops as a result of this movement. The cord and placenta contribute in no way to the baby's nourishment; neither does the menstrual blood which collects in the womb during pregnancy. The dirty blood, swallowed inadvertently by the child, colors its first feces black. Until the fifth month he grows solely by the will of God; during that month he begins to feed through a conduit running from his mother's stomach to her uterus. At the same time the baby begins to breathe. Air from its mother's lungs enters the baby's nose and mouth, goes to its lungs, and finally reaches the blood stream, where it acts as the force that drives the blood. The baby does not excrete in the womb. Everything it eats turns into blood to fuel its growth.

As the months pass, the baby's body alternates between hard and soft. The village midwife estimates how far a pregnancy has progressed by feeling the baby's hardness as well as its size and the height of the uterus, an estimate which is often at odds with that of the government midwife. Both subscribe to the theory that a seven month fetus (whose body is hard) has a better chance for survival than an eight month fetus (who has become soft again).

PENEMPAH BIDAN AND LENGGANG PERUT

In the seventh month of pregnancy, the prospective mother and her family present the bidan of their choice with a dollar or two and some sireh leaves (*Piper betel*), pinang nuts (*Areca catechu*), gambier (*Uncaria gambir*) and slaked lime, the ingredients of betel quids. A midwife reserved in this manner (*penempah bidan*) is ideally obliged to stay in her patient's vicinity when her anticipated time of delivery nears (Chen 1974–1975:337; Chen 1975: 103). In actuality, however, she does not keep close track of her clients' due dates, but goes about her daily activities until alerted that a patient is in active labor. Sapiah, the most popular bidan in

[86]

Merchang, earned the better part of her income tapping rubber. If notified that a patient was in labor before she left for her morning's work, she examined the pregnant woman, and if birth was imminent remained at her patient's side. If all seemed normal, but labor promised to be prolonged, she reassured the family that she would return from the morning's tapping in plenty of time to assist in the baby's birth. In the past, when women worked closer to their homes, a reserved bidan would have been easily accessible to her clients at all times of day. Within recent years, rubber tapping and cash cropping of tobacco and watermelon have taken agricultural workers further from their homes. Since Sapiah's husband did not earn enough to support her family, she could not afford to stay home idle as each patient neared her due date, and often spent the morning at remote work places. If a woman went into labor while Sapiah was tapping rubber or working on her tobacco farm, another bidan had to be called in. The reserved bidan is not obliged to return the penempah, whether she is present at the delivery or not. However, a bidan who has not been reserved (*bidan tarik*, a "pulled-in" midwife) is entitled to a higher fee.

A first pregnancy requires special rites to ensure ease of labor and safety of delivery. Traditionally, the reserved midwife performed the ceremony of *lenggang perut* (rocking the abdomen) during the seventh month of the first pregnancy, a ritual that is rapidly becoming rarer and more abbreviated, due in large measure to censure by the Office of Religious Affairs (see Mahmud Salim 1975). Many clients prefer to retain only those parts, such as the *lepas* (a ritual action signifying passage out of a dangerous state), that they feel are absolutely essential. Others request Islamic prayers and water used for ablutions at the mosque to be substituted for traditional forms.

A full-scale lenggang perut, such as one I was fortunate enough to observe, requires elaborate preparations. The assembled women mixed rice flour and water to make neutralizing rice

[87]

paste (*tepung tawar*) to counteract the spirits' noxious influence by balancing their heat and air with its cooling qualities of earth and water (see chap. 3). Small green limes (*limau nipis*) were squeezed into bath water to decrease spiritual heat further.

The women threaded turmeric, *jeringau* (*Acorus calamus*, the sweet flag), and *cikur* (*Kaemferia galanga*) on a string. Cikur and jeringau, used to soothe a baby's fever, are employed here for the protection of the fetus. Turmeric's royal yellow color frightens the spirits because it reminds them of their defeat at the hands of King Solomon, putative ancestor of all Malay royalty.

They placed some coins in a plate, covered them with raw rice and added a coconut. A length of cord, knotted and looped around the nut, completed the *keras*. This ritual object is an indispensable part of childbirth and healing ceremonies. The coconut, with its liquid and solid contents, is a stand-in for the pregnant uterus. Its hairiness and suggestion of a face also make it a double for the human head. The cord looped around the coconut symbolizes the umbilical cord and is, as well, an essential part of the lepas.

When all the preparations had been completed, the young mother-to-be removed all her clothing except her sarong. She lay on a mat while the bidan felt her bare abdomen to determine whether the baby was positioned properly, head down and body vertical. Seven cloths of different colors were placed beneath the patient. Quickly, the bidan and the woman's mother, sitting on either side of her, tied each cloth in turn loosely over her belly, rocked her gently, untied the cloth, and pulled it out from under her. Each release of a cloth signified the release of the mother from spiritual danger. One after the other, the bidan rolled three plants across the pregnant belly: Palas leaves, used to tie rice seedlings; leaves of the areca palm, employed to brush noxious spiritual influences away from the afflicted; and a joint of bamboo, one end open and the other closed, a duplicate of the womb's anatomy. After rolling the coconut three times around the

[88]

woman's body, the bidan placed it on her abdomen and pretended to cleave it with a *parang* (like a machete). The symbolic release of its contents is meant to encourage the successful release of the contents of the womb.

When this part of the lenggang perut was over, the midwife bathed her patient in lime juice and water, to which she added the neutralizing rice paste. She placed a spot of rice paste on the woman's forehead and her own, and tied the herbal string around her patient's waist. She touched a razor blade to the girl's forehead, arms and feet to harden her *semangat* (vital forces) and to act as a deterrent to spirits, who are frightened of all sharp objects, especially those made of iron.

Three times the bidan released the mother-to-be from the dangers of pregnancy: First, by the untying of double slipknots in long strips of palm leaves (called *pelepas*, that which releases), pulled apart at the climatic moment of a jampi; next, by passing the keras' looped cord over her head to her feet, as a baby passes through the birth canal; and finally, by utilizing the cord, into which rice from the keras had been inserted, to toss the rice in her direction as a second jampi ended.

After she had dressed, the woman was presented with a large bowl of *nasi semangat*, bright yellow glutinous rice cooked in coconut cream and decorated with red hardboiled eggs and paper flowers. Nasi semangat (life-force rice) is eaten at weddings, circumcisions, and other important occasions, to strengthen the life-force of those who eat it. The eggs, symbolic of birth, denote a change of status. After the pregnant woman ate one of the eggs and a token amount of nasi semangat, the bidan performed the last lepas. Her unloosening of a final slipknot ended the ceremony. The participants and their guests sat down to a kenduri of nasi semangat and fish curry. All the guests were given packages of nasi semangat and a colored egg to take home. The bidan was given ten coconuts and a sarong as well.

The lenggang perut is usually performed only for a first preg-

[89]

nancy, since the woman is not yet pandai (adept) at carrying and delivering her babies. If she has a stillbirth, the ritual may be repeated during a subsequent pregnancy.

DANGERS DURING PREGNANCY

Pregnancy, in Merchang, is considered a normal condition, requiring few changes in a woman's daily life. Regular physical activity is believed to facilitate labor, and most women work until well into the third trimester. The diet, on the whole, does not change during pregnancy. Except for being cautious about eating much jackfruit and durian during the early months when it is feared the fetal blood clot might be liquified, women follow no dietary rules or recommendations specific to pregnancy. The normal diet, they feel, is sufficient for both the mother and the growing baby. Most women throw away the vitamins given out at the government midwife's clinic since they consider them unnecessary and possibly harmful. Their bitter taste may be an indication of their "heat," and their potency may cause the baby to grow so large that he tears the birth canal on his way into the world.

Women in many Southeast Asian cultures are expected to have occasional food cravings during pregnancy. In some parts of the Philippines, unsatisfied cravings are feared to cause a miscarriage or deform the fetus (Hart et al. 1965:34−40). Thais believe a frustrated mother will drool uncontrollably (Hart et al. 1965: 129). In Trengganu, it is the baby, rather than the mother, who runs the risk of drooling, since it is he who really craves the food. The mother only acts as the baby's agent. A bidan told me a story to illustrate the point:

> Long ago, a man grew an enormous jackfruit which he meant to present to the rajah. On his way to the palace, he passed a pregnant woman, who looked at the fruit with longing and begged a piece from him. Although he worried that the rajah might not accept an imperfect gift, he broke off a piece and gave it to the woman to eat. When he

[90]

reached the palace, his fears were realized. The rajah was offended when he noticed the empty section of the jackfruit. "I gave it to the child within the woman's womb," said the man, "for it was the babe who requested it." The rajah refused to believe him, and ordered his men to bring the woman before him. He took his *keris* and ripped open her belly. Inside sat the baby, chewing on a piece of jackfruit.

Village midwives who have attended meetings at the district capital Health Center are aware of the symptoms of hypertension and the toxemias of pregnancy. They recognize that placental retention and postpartum hemorrhage are potentially life-threatening and may require the speedy removal of a patient to the General Hospital. Aside from these, dangers during pregnancy are considered less likely to affect a mother than her unborn child. Danger to the baby ranges from minor transient conditions to deformity and death.

According to English observers around the turn of the century (Clifford 1898:48−51; Skeat 1972:348−50; Maxwell 1881:19), both the father and mother-to-be were obliged to follow numerous taboos to ensure that the child would be born physically perfect and lacking undesirable personality traits, and that the mother would not die in childbirth. During his wife's pregnancy, a husband could not cut his hair, sit on his doorstep, or do harm to any living creature. If he passed the night at the home of a friend whose wife was also expecting a baby, he had to remain there for two nights before returning home or his own wife would die. "Why would she die?" asks Mr. Clifford. "God alone knows, but such is the teaching of the men of old, the wise ones of ancient days." The expectant mother, for her part, was forbidden to sleep during the day, for fear of evil spirits. She should be careful to say nothing mocking about man or beast, lest her baby be born with the very qualities she disparaged. She supposedly lived in fear of a lunar eclipse, which "brought unnamed terrors in its wake."[10] (Clifford 1898:51). The theme running through these accounts is that of blind unquestioning obedience to prescriptions and proscriptions which, if not followed, were feared to result invariably in grave consequences for mother and/or child. This view is echoed by recent scholarship. According to Colson, "the consequences of most pantang violations are considered to be a certainty" (1971:34). He cites as pantang (a word often glossed as taboo) with the highest degree of adherence, such examples as, "The husband of a pregnant woman should not shoot a beast in the eye or the child *will* be born blind," and "The husband of a pregnant woman may not pull on the legs of any dead animal or the child *will* have one leg shorter than the other" (1971:149, emphasis added). These, and many other birth pantang cited by Colson, are in the form of a cause and effect relationship: if one does something, certain consequences invariably follow. Whyte (1974:64) carries it one step further. He says, "In Indonesia and Malaya, the father should not kill or wound any animal during his wife's pregnancy or the child will be wounded in the same way. This affects the protein intake of the entire family." Since fishing not only provides almost all the animal protein in the Malay diet, but is also an important part of the Malaysian economy, such a belief would not only affect a family's nutrition adversely, but would be disastrous for the economy as a whole. Whyte's conclusion, although it logically follows from his preceding statement, presupposes that Malay belief is monolithic, invariable, and therefore strictly acted out.

In actuality, I found that Malay beliefs in general, and birth pantang in particular, have built-in flexibility. Neglect of them is usually fastened upon as an ex post facto explanation of why some abnormal or unpleasant event has occurred. Most pantang can hardly be called taboos, since they are neither implicitly obeyed, nor do they carry a certain punishment for their nonobservance, either through human or supernatural agencies. They are often such practical-sounding advice as admonitions to pregnant women not to sleep during the day or heat may collect in their cheeks and make them swell, or not to sit on a chair, instead of the floor, as their ankles may swell. Other pantang reflect belief in sympathetic magic. Mothers are cautioned that tying cloths around their throats or arms may cause the umbilical cord to loop itself about the baby's throat. Fathers are warned that sitting on their house steps and blocking the entrance may obstruct their wife's birth canal during delivery. Mothers are told that bathing in the evening may mean that their babies will be born with excessive amniotic fluid (see McArthur 1962:23 for similar observations in other states of Malaysia). In spite of such warnings, I have observed prospective parents exhibit all these behaviors. While the neighbors might think such people are tempting fate, their chances of escaping unscathed are considered good. It is only because the "rules" are not implicitly obeyed that satisfying ex post facto explanations are possible.[11]

The prohibitions of childbirth, such as those pertaining to the slaughter of animals by a father-to-be, are often both practical and flexible. These birth pantang in no way restrict the family's usual economic activities or dietary intake, since neither fishing nor the ordinary slaughter of chickens is prohibited. Other pantang are equally practical: the husband of a pregnant woman should not hammer nails into wood lest his wife have a difficult labor, *unless he is a carpenter*. Again, the pantang is conditional and allows for the continuation of normal daily life.

Although slaughter of domestic animals for the purpose of eating them is not believed to harm the unborn child, deliberately injuring an animal might. For example, cutting off the claws of a crab or the toes of a chicken may cause the child to be born with its digits short or missing. The important word is "may." The outcome is by no means certain. Usually nothing will happen to the baby, but if something should, its parents can explain their child's deformity or illness by referring to an incident which occurred during its mother's pregnancy.

The husband of one of my neighbors amused himself by hitting stray cats and dogs, and had actually killed one during his wife's first pregnancy. After she was delivered of a stillbirth, the tragedy was ascribed to her husband's cruel treatment of the animals. When I heard she was pregnant again, I remarked that I supposed her husband was now being very scrupulous about his behavior. "Oh, no," she said. "He still hits the animals, just as he always did." Luckily this pregnancy ended with the birth of a healthy boy, denying the neighbors the pleasure of nodding their heads wisely about the father having gotten his just deserts once more.

To avoid an increased risk to the unborn, animals must be slaughtered cleanly and for good cause. This pantang extends as well to the cutting of wood. It cannot be an act of wanton destruction, and the father-to-be must make sure he leaves no jagged edges or splinters. Animals and wood possess semangat, the life-force that permeates the universe and dwells in man, beast, plant, and rock (cf. Endicott 1970). All share a form of life: the life of a fire is swift and soon burns out; a rock's life is slow, long, and dreamlike. Slashing and splintering wood is equivalent to cutting and chopping an animal's flesh and bones. Both are equated with the baby's disfigurement, since all are bound up in the actions of the father, the baby's primary source of life. The father's actions exert their strongest influence during the earliest months, before the baby's form has been defined. His influence continues throughout pregnancy, lessening as the months go by and ceasing when the umbilical cord is cut. Even minor actions, such as forgetting to untie a bundle promptly, may bring harm to the unborn. To lower the odds, a father must remember his wife's condition at all times. If he recalls the existence of his unborn child while he is involved in a questionable activity, and says, "Wake up Missy or Sonny, don't be startled and be harmed by this" (*Bangun Mek Awang, jangan terkejut kena badi*), he may avert the danger.

A mother's being startled or disgusted during pregnancy may harm her child. Besides providing ex post facto explanations for

[94]

infantile abnormalities, this Malay theory of prenatal influence (*lekat kenan*, or sticking birth defect) can also suggest a cure. If a newborn spits up excessively and its mother remembers being startled by seeing a cat vomit during her pregnancy, she can clip some fur, claws and whiskers from the cat, burn them, and mark the child with the ashes. If a baby alarms its parents by thrashing about like a chicken in the throes of death, the mother, attributing its behavior to her disgust at seeing a chicken slaughtered, will burn some feathers for the treatment.[12] These home remedies usually suffice, but if the condition persists the bidan may recommend that a bomoh be called in for consultation and treatment. It may be necessary to transfer the illness, which exits by way of the baby's toes upon the recitation of a jampi, to a rice paste figurine of the culprit animal, placed at the infant's feet. The infected figurine is later tossed into the underbrush, where it cannot inflict harm.[13]

Serious defects, such as missing joints, cannot be cured and must be accepted as lessons (not punishments) from God. The lesson is twofold and clear: remember your wife and child when they are most vulnerable; and be careful not to inflict unnecessary cruelty on animals. Those who follow these lessons not only obey the teachings of Mohammad, but also avoid possible contamination from badi.

Wilkinson (1959:62) calls badi "the ghostly influences haunting a scene of slaughter." Von de Wall (quoted in Skeat 1972:427) describes it as "the enchanting or destroying influence which issues from anything, e.g., from a tiger which one sees, from a poison-tree which one passes under, from the saliva of a mad dog, from an action which one has performed; the contagious principle of morbid matter." Skeat (1972:427) says "badi is the name given to the evil principle which, according to the view of Malay medicine men, attends (like an evil angel) everything that has life, including trees, stones and minerals." East coast bomoh are much more specific concerning the nature of badi. It is only resident in

[95]

recent human corpses, or in animals, especially wild ones.

Hunting at any time is dangerous. Its danger is heightened considerably when one's wife is pregnant. Killing domestic animals and fish is a necessary part of village life and carries no risk if done humanely. Chickens belong to the world of man—the cultivated, domesticated, familiar kampung. Fish, although wild, are essential to the diet, and fishing is the primary occupation of many villagers. Hunting is a nonessential activity which takes a man out of the protection of the kampung and into the jungle, where dangers range from savage animals to untamed spirits. As frightening as the hantu of the village and fields might be, the jungle spirits are known to be wilder, more unpredictable, unused to the ways of men and resentful of their encroachment.[14] The animals of the jungle are cherished by the spirits, particularly wild counterparts of domestic species, such as the jungle fowl, the wild goat (serow) and three kinds of deer: the large *rusa*, the smaller *kijang*, and the tiny *pelanduk* or *kancil* (mouse deer). Killing these animals can expose the hunter, and by extension his unborn child, to the wrath of their ghostly friends and to the malign influence of the animals' badi (also known as *jinggi* and *kuwung*), which is released at the time of their death.

The badi of human corpses can be extremely dangerous to the unborn, to infants, whose semangat has not yet become strong, and to people whose semangat has been weakened. Prospective parents, and sick or delicate people, may have an unpleasant aftermath to a visit of consolation. An adult with depleted semangat may become ill, or his previous illness may be aggravated. The unborn child may be afflicted with *badi mayat* (badi of a human corpse), which manifests itself as a wasting disease. The baby refuses to eat, takes on the appearance of a corpse, and dies within weeks of its birth. Considering the severity of badi mayat, if Malays believed in a direct cause and effect relationship, it would be simple common sense for all persons in a vulnerable category to stay away from the dead. That they do not is, once again, a sign

[96]

that the belief is one of increased probabilities rather than certainties, and that the peril is remote enough for many people to test the limits or flirt with danger. Badi mayat, like the more benign varieties of lekat kenan, is an ex post facto explanation. Unlike lekat kenan, which provides a cure as well as an explanation for what seem to be, on the whole, self-limiting conditions, a diagnosis of badi mayat may actually be a self-fulfilling prophecy.

A diagnosis of badi mayat was a contributory factor in the death of Rohani's baby. She had been a large and healthy child, weighing eight pounds at birth, but after a month she began to cry when put to the breast and refused to nurse. She was changed to bottle feeding and given prepared baby cereal to eat, but only accepted small amounts of food, slept most of the time and became limp and listless. At five weeks she looked gaunt and drawn. She cried weakly and coughed frequently. I persuaded Rohani and her mother to let me drive them and the baby to the nearest Health Center. As a precautionary measure against further illness, the grandmother chewed a quid of betel and painted her bright red saliva on the baby's forehead, nose and cheeks. This, she said, would make the baby unattractive to hantu.

Unfortunately, the doctor, who came to the Center one morning a week, was unavailable. The Hospital Assistant on duty quickly examined the baby's chest and prescribed cough medicine. I was unsatisfied with his diagnosis and treatment, and proposed to take them to see a pediatrician at the General Hospital in Kuala Trengganu the following day. When we reached home, after the visit to the Health Center, my car stalled at the bottom of the hill leading to Rohani's house. As she walked up the hill, carrying the baby, dozens of people who had not previously seen the child were appalled at her corpselike appearance. They all agreed that she had badi mayat. Rohani's mother reminded her of the time, early in her pregnancy, when she was startled by the sight of a young cousin's corpse.

They stopped at the house of a bomoh along the way, to ask

[97]

what could be done for the sick child. His diagnosis was more hopeful. Although the baby was beginning to look like a corpse, her complexion was not pale and waxy. Therefore her problem was not caused by badi mayat but by *sambang* (a condition which may occur when a baby is born with the umbilical cord looped around its neck). When this occurs, the bidan quickly unwraps the cord and does an immediate lepas (ritual release), followed by another lepas three days later and a third at the end of the postpartum period. Usually this is enough to take the baby out of the state of danger. In the Malay cosmos, however, nothing is certain for good or for ill. What worked in the past may not work at any particular time, each bomoh's magical knowledge is limited, magic itself is fallible, disease states vary in intensity, and people vary in their physical and spiritual resistance. Most important, the curer must be in harmony (*sesuai*) with the patient for a cure to be successful.

Sambang can be fatal. Instead of growing plumper, a baby who has sambang becomes progressively thinner and finally dies if its condition is untreated. The bomoh further diagnosed the baby as suffering from *sakit meroyan*, caused by a hantu which arises from the afterbirth, the amniotic fluid and the blood of parturition. The bidan's precautions usually prevent the hantu meroyan from harming the mother and child. Occasionally, however, due to the midwife's incompetence, or any of the other reasons mentioned above, it can cause serious trouble. Sakit meroyan afflicts the mother with postpartum blues. In its most virulent form, it turns into postpartum psychosis, causing a mother to reject her baby and even attempt to kill it. Babies suffering from sakit meroyan refuse the breast and cry night and day. Weakness brought on by sambang increases a baby's vulnerability to sakit meroyan. The two conditions in tandem produce a synergistic, and sinister, effect.

The bomoh advised Rohani first to change her baby's name to another more harmonious (sesuai) with her personality. The

[98]

discordance set up by a "wrong" name may contribute to a child's vulnerability. Many children in Merchang are known by two names: a school name (the one on their birth certificates) and a home name (given to them for reasons of health). The bomoh recites a series of names while dropping grains of rice into a glass of water. The wrong name causes the rice to drop to the bottom of the glass. Three grains of rice floating on the top are an indication that the right name has been chosen.

A name change is often all a child needs to improve its health, however, Rohani's baby's condition called for stronger measures. The family made a keras, similar to the one used for lenggang perut, of coins, rice, and a coconut, but instead of raw cord, seven joined pieces of white thread and seven of yellow were coiled atop the coconut. The bomoh explained that the white cord represented the baby's *urat* [15] and the yellow her blood. [16] In imitation of the birth process, he passed the looped threads over the baby's head and drew them down her body until they dropped from her feet, first the white and then the yellow. Reborn in this manner, with a new name, perhaps the baby would have a second chance at life.

When the spiritual prophylaxis had been accomplished, I suggested that now it might be wise to visit the pediatrician. Although the baby's semangat had been strengthened, her body was still weak. At the very least, the hospital could supply Rohani with vitamins. I thought this would be a convincing argument, since Malays have great faith in the strengthening powers of vitamin pills. I convinced a village midwife, who accompanied me to Rohani's house to speak to her husband. Although the bidan added her voice to mine, saying that everything possible must be done for a sick baby, hospital medicine as well as village medicine, the father did not think it necessary for his baby to visit the hospital immediately. If, over the next month, she did not improve as a result of the bomoh's treatment, there would be time enough to try something else.

[99]

The baby continued to waste away, and people began to question the bomoh's diagnosis. Since the treatments for sambang and sakit meroyan did not improve the baby's condition, the likelihood grew in the minds of many that their original opinion was correct—that the baby was suffering from badi mayat. A second bomoh privately questioned the first bomoh's competence. If he had been handling the case, he would first have transferred the sickness to a rice paste figurine and then advised the parents to take the baby to the hospital. Unless the underlying spiritual causes are removed, hospital medicine is useless, but for purely physical conditions it is frequently stronger and faster than village medicine. For such a severe case, he said, it was imperative to treat both body and spirit with the strongest means available.

Medical ethics and Malay courtesy prevented the bomoh from volunteering any advice. Rohani's husband did not call on this second bomoh, nor did he heed the midwife's advice. The baby's condition progressively deteriorated. Two weeks after our visit to the Health Center, the parents brought the baby to my house and asked me to drive the mother and child to the hospital. The baby was shrunken and her head looked like a skull. When we reached the hospital I asked Rohani to wait while I persuaded the pediatrician to see them right away. The usual hospital procedure involves a wait for several hours to see a resident. If the resident thinks that a further examination by a specialist is in order, the patient must wait again, or return for another appointment. From the looks of the baby, there was no time to waste. By the time I returned to the waiting area to tell Rohani the pediatrician would see the baby at once, she had been surrounded by a crowd of fellow patients. They assured her that since the baby had badi mayat there was no point in seeing a doctor. He wouldn't understand her condition or know how to treat it. I pulled them away from the crowd, to the pediatrician's office. He diagnosed the baby as severely dehydrated due to gastroenteritis, and ordered an immediate transfusion. I left them in the pediatric ward, hoping that the treatment had been started in time to save the child. Early the next morning I was awakened by Rohani's husband. He asked me to bring home his wife and baby. The child had died during the night. Her weight at death was four and one-half pounds, close to half her birth weight. The family would have preferred to have the baby die at home, but they did not blame the hospital for her death. They thought the transfusion must have been too strong for such a small child, but the baby was doomed and would have died anyway.

THE CULTURAL MAPPING OF PREGNANCY

In contrast to the strange terrain in which many pregnant American women find themselves—dependent upon books and classes to guide them to their destination—conception and gestation are well-mapped territories to rural Malays. Cultural signposts furnish parents with information about the advantages and risks of following subsidiary paths ("rules to break rules") or even leaving the highroad altogether. The mapping of contingencies, in particular, is an adaptive strategy for dealing with the uncertainties and disasters of birth.

Malay theories of prenatal influence do not make pregnancy a time of high anxiety, as earlier observers believed. Although there are many admonitions regarding behavior at this time, they are often observed in the breach. Probably nothing bad will come of it anyhow, people reason, but if it should, there will be time enough to deal with it then. A diagnosis of lekat kenan, when it concerns minor transitory conditions, reduces anxiety since the diagnosis often provides the cure. Worried parents are presented with a simple course of action, relieving them of the corrosive feeling of impotence, and the treatment actually "works," since these self-limiting conditions would ameliorate or disappear even if nothing were done.

The dark side of these concepts is that they can lead to theories

[101]

that can inhibit the discovery process (Alland 1970:52). A diagnosis of badi mayat may be a death sentence for a baby, since it reduces the chance that parents will seek appropriate medical care. But, although diagnoses of sambang, sakit meroyan, and badi mayat, based on false notions of causality, are "bad" theories in an adaptive sense, it would be incorrect to say that they, by themselves, caused the death of Rohani's baby. These folk diagnoses were not made until after the baby's first contact with hospital-based medicine. It was the combination of one imperfectly learned medical system (on the part of the Hospital Assistant) and another whose theory and practice, in this case, were faulty (on the part of the bomoh and villagers) which proved deadly for the child.

· 5 ·

Government Midwife and
Traditional Midwife

Around the turn of the century, Englishmen in Malaya were collecting vast quantities of data on "the folklore of uncivilised races" (Blagden in Skeat 1972:xi). Childbirth customs were described at length as examples of primitive superstition; the midwife's practical role was neglected in favor of her ritual activity. To Annandale and Robinson, the chief duties of the bidan "consist in reciting charms to scare away the Earth Spirits" (1903–1904:63). Skeat (1972), Winstedt (1920), and Wilkinson (1908) were interested in the methods she employed for the selection of a lucky place for the birth, and the measures she used for spiritual prophylaxis.

The midwife's practice may have made fascinating reading for Edwardian England, but it was not supposed to be of any real assistance to the benighted natives. Sir Hugh Clifford, in fact, considered her a malign influence on women in labor. He depicted pregnancy as a time of superstitious fear and numerous taboos, and childbirth as "a day when [the female character in his story] nearly loses her life by reason of the barbarities which Malay science considers necessary if a woman is to win through her confinement without mishap" (1898:51).

[103]

Attitudes toward Malay traditional birth attendants of those who think in terms of Western medical practice have changed little over the years. Articles meant for medical professionals and social scientists concentrate on "superstitious customs surrounding childbirth" (e.g., Wylde 1956) and argue that indigenous medical practices are "not only directly responsible for ill-health by prescribing the wrong things for conditions that are quite normal, e.g., pregnancy, but by getting in the way of modern medicine . . . indirectly prevent good health" (Siti Hasmah 1968: 16). Although medical writers occasionally applaud the reassurance the village midwife gives her patients, they condemn her purportedly brutal and unsanitary techniques as contributing to neonatal tetanus (Chen 1976) and rupture of the uterus (Chen 1974–1975; Siti Hasmah 1968:6; Sambhi 1968:347; Thambu 1971:294).

Although the Malaysian medical establishment is virtually unanimous in its disapproval of the traditional midwife, an uneasy truce exists between the representatives of the two traditions.[1] The services of the bidan kampung are indispensable at this time. Traditional birth attendants conduct half of all deliveries in rural areas (which themselves constitute 54 percent of all deliveries in Malaysia (Country Report 1975:13). One of the reasons for this is the lack of institutionally trained personnel. Government midwives, because of their heavy workloads, may not be available to respond to a call because they are attending to another delivery, or are off duty or on leave (Siti Hasmah 1975a:2). If patients were unable to secure the help of a bidan kampung, some would be obliged to give birth unattended. Besides being sought after as emergency substitutes, traditional midwives are often called in preference to, or in conjunction with, government midwives since they offer many services considered essential by their clients that government midwives do not include in their duties, such as postnatal massage, housekeeping help, and ritual expertise.

[104]

Although the village midwife's current utility is undeniable, her days appear to be numbered. Under the Midwives Act of 1966, and the Registration Regulation of 1971, traditional midwives are required to register with the Midwives Board as "Untrained Midwives" before they are allowed to practice. The closing date of registration was July 31, 1972. As some of these midwives were then more than seventy years old, and only 38 percent were younger than sixty, it is estimated that Malay traditional birth attendants will slowly be phased out over the next twenty to thirty years and gradually replaced by government midwives. During this phase, the Ministry of Health hopes that the village midwife will increasingly relinquish her obstetric practices, which it deems harmful, while retaining her services as housekeeper and masseuse and, ideally, joining the government midwife as part of a team:

> While discouraging new recruits from rendering traditional midwifery, every effort is now being made to utilize the existing kampung bidans as motivators of health and diverting their skills to a more harmless service to rural mothers. [Siti Hasmah 1975*b*:5]

Condemnation of the bidan's activities comes, as well, from the Islamic religious establishment. Her dealings with the supernatural in general, and her performance of lenggang perut in particular, have been denounced as disturbing vestiges of Hindu customs which threaten Islamic integrity (Mahmud Salim 1975). The bidan kampung is thus in the curious position of being an amateur and interloper in the view of the establishment while being considered a medical expert and distinguished member of the community by her fellow villagers.

How harmful are the traditional midwife's practices, and to what extent do they differ from those of the government midwife? Upon what can we base our estimation of her performance? Recent accounts of rural Malay childbirth come from McArthur (1962); Strange (1971); Djamour (1966), who witnessed at least

[105]

one delivery, and Chen (1973, 1974–1975, 1975), who did not. Chen's material is by far the most detailed, but since, as he remarks, "Modesty prohibits men other than her husband, her father and the bomoh to be present in the [delivery] room," it must be taken as hearsay evidence rather than the account of an observer. The ethnological record is overly dependent on data obtained from informant interviews, or from accounts by earlier authors based on information compiled in a similar fashion. In contrast, as an apprentice to a bidan kampung, I observed and assisted in dozens of deliveries and was instructed in the ritual, obstetrical, and nursing practices that are the duties of the traditional Malay birth attendant. I also formed a working relationship with the government midwife which enabled me, in return for providing nighttime transportation, to attend her antenatal clinic and to be present on occasions when she supervised deliveries. In this chapter I compare the training, antenatal care, and social role of the government and village midwives. In the following chapter I will discuss the traditional midwife as a ritual and a medical practitioner, and then compare her procedures in the latter role with those of the government midwife.

THE GOVERNMENT MIDWIFE

Before a government midwife is posted to her first assignment, she has been instructed in general anatomy and physiology, management of normal labor and puerperium, symptoms suggesting departure from the normal, and the keeping of records (Chen 1975:134–135). Her two years of training include eighteen months in the hospital, during which time she attends at least thirty women in labor and witnesses not less than twenty deliveries (Rosina 1975:3).

Besides holding a weekly antenatal clinic, the government midwife is expected to visit cases at home at least four times prior to delivery (Halimah 1975:2). She must be on call throughout the

[106]

day and night to attend to women in labor, seven days a week. During weekends she may leave her station only with the permission of the nursing sister in charge (Chen 1975:147). She is required to make home visits daily for the first ten days after delivery, and again on the twentieth and fortieth days following birth (Chen 1975:159). These requirements, at least in Merchang, are an ideal striven toward but never attained.[2]

The government midwife in charge of the mukim of Merchang, who I will call Halimah, had recently been assigned to the area as her first post. She was a childless young woman in her early twenties. Both she and her husband, a middle-echelon government employee, came from west coast states. Their education and standard of living far exceeded those of most of the local inhabitants. Halimah's husband owned one of the few cars in the vicinity. The government provided her with a motor scooter that allowed her to perform her duties within an area three to four times larger than that of the village midwives, none of whom owned so much as a bicycle.

Halimah's relations with the villagers and the various traditional midwives were complex and equivocal. She was always pleasant and smiling, and avoided open conflict whenever possible, in the best Malay tradition of correct behavior. Halimah told me that when she first came to Merchang she was grateful for the friendship of Sapiah, the most active bidan kampung, who was willing to teach Halimah from her wealth of practical knowledge and long years of experience. This pupil-teacher dyad, the traditional method of instructing a novice bidan kampung, could not continue for long because of the authority conflict inherent in the relationship. Halimah had the weight of the government behind her and the authority of institutional training, while Sapiah had the authority that comes from being the descendant of a long line of bidan, personally inheriting the necessary qualifications, and conducting a successful practice for more than thirty years. Neither could be happy in a subordinate position. As Halimah's

[107]

practical expertise increased, she became more secure in her assumption of authority. When both midwives were in attendance, it was Halimah who conducted the actual delivery. Surface relationships, as always, remained cordial, but a good deal of resentment rose to the surface when Halimah was not present.

The villagers respected Halimah for her education, official authority, command of scientific apparatus and medicines and, especially, for the ability to call for an ambulance in case of emergency. The only reliable means of communicating with the General Hospital is located at the police station. There are no private telephones, and the one public pay phone was out of order more often than not. To request such aid of the police was beyond the courage of most villagers. Ambulances were dispatched only in the case of life-threatening or severely acute conditions, and frequently took as long as four hours to arrive in Merchang, since they served a large area and might be out on calls.

The villagers' admiration for Halimah as a representative of scientific medicine did not extend to her as a person. They considered her a foreigner who didn't understand the local dialect and spoke Malay with a west coast accent. Her higher class position made them uncomfortable. Their feeling that the government midwife was an outsider was shared, as well, by Halimah and her husband, who hoped to go to America for further study which would assure their advancement and posting somewhere more to their liking. Halimah considered the people of Merchang ignorant, dirty, and behind the times. Nevertheless, she made some accommodations to their beliefs. She washed the afterbirth and prepared it for traditional burial. She did not interfere with the rituals of village midwives or the families of parturient women, or criticize such acts in their presence. Although these beliefs were alien to Halimah, she was sensitive to her patients' feelings.

Aside from their discomfort at her foreign ways and superior class position, many villagers felt that most of the government midwife's services were superfluous, merely duplicating those of the more experienced village midwives. Still, they felt that as citizens of Malaysia they were entitled to the full measure of her services. They were extremely resentful if she did not come when called or if she took an hour or so to arrive. Women who gave birth while her antenatal clinic was in progress had to do without her services. She asked the village midwives not to call her between midnight and 6 A.M. since she was afraid of traveling alone at night. It was this fear that provided the impetus for our relationship when I offered to drive her to night calls.

Halimah rarely made visits to homes in Kg. Durian Pahit and was never present at a birth in this jungle outpost hamlet. The mud and stick road that the villagers erected over the padi field required goat-footed agility at the best of times. During the monsoon season, the kampung was completely inaccessible except by boat. Halimah, knowing that she would not assist at their deliveries, supplied her patients from Durian Pahit with medicines to disinfect the baby's umbilical stump and to relieve the mother's afterpains, when they came to her antenatal clinic during the last month of pregnancy. Even so, they complained bitterly behind her back and wanted to prepare a petition to her superiors, but they never did. Halimah made her own complaint to the authorities about the condition of the road and its interference with her duties. In 1979, two years after she left Merchang, a new paved road was constructed, linking Kg. Durian Pahit with the rest of the mukim.

Villagers frequently compared Halimah to their previous government midwife, Zainab, a native of Trengganu. They said that Halimah was lazy, and that she made fewer home visits than they had been accustomed to receiving. A comparison of the number of times each government midwife was reported by villagers to have made home visits, however, shows that Halimah's record was considerably better than that of her predecessor (see table 8). Preference for a local woman, rather than actual performance, was the basis for this criticism.

[109]

TABLE 8

HOME VISITS OF GOVERNMENT MIDWIVES IN MERCHANG
(A survey of four kampung, whose population represents approximately
half of the families under their supervision)

Halimah

Antenatal				Postnatal		
No.	*%*			*No.*	*%*	
0	26	(9)		0	26	(9)
1	29	(10)		1	31	(11)
2	17	(6)		2	14	(5)
3	20	(7)		3	17	(6)
4	6	(2)		4	3	(1)
5	0			5	3	(1)
6	3	(1)		6	3	(1)
				7	3	(1)

N = 35

Zainab

Antenatal				Postnatal		
No.	*%*			*No.*	*%*	
0	60	(15)		0	24	(6)
1	4	(1)		1	28	(7)
2	20	(5)		2	16	(4)
3	8	(2)		3	20	(5)
4	8	(2)		4	12	(3)

N = 25

THE VILLAGE MIDWIVES

Six village midwives were in active practice in the area covered
by the government midwife. Three others assisted at occasional
deliveries, and one woman, who had lost most of one foot because

[110]

of diabetic gangrene, was now employed only as an adjunct to the government midwife, performing the rituals of childbirth, clean-up after delivery, and massage of the new mother.

All the active midwives, women in their late fifties to seventies, claimed to have been in practice for thirty years or more, follow-ing a long apprenticeship with their mothers. The latest in a long line of bidan kampung, they were considered to have inherited the talent and bravery necessary to practice their skills.

Of the three who were relatively inactive, one was a woman in her thirties. Her neighbors considered her rather young for the job and called her only if an older bidan was not available or could not be reached in time to attend an imminent birth. Another, a woman in her fifties, was not popular because she was suspected of harboring a *pelesit*, a familiar spirit that makes its "mother" appear fascinating to the opposite sex in return for meals of eggs or, some say, blood. Although most people considered her singu-larly unattractive, they pointed out that her husband showed no signs of deserting her. The pelesit was evidently holding up its end of the bargain, since it was plain that her husband saw her with enchanted eyes. Unfortunately, pelesit enjoy making chil-dren cry, a sure sign of their presence, one of my neighbors told me. Her youngest child always cried whenever this woman ap-proached. More serious than that, pelesit may interfere with the normal progress of birth. It is easy to see why calls upon this woman's services were rare.

The third relatively inactive bidan was a great rarity among Malay traditional birth attendants: a man.[3] Pak Su Zali, the headman (*ketua kampung*) of Kg. Durian Pahit, was a famous masseur, and the son of a bidan. Because of the hamlet's isolation, he attended all deliveries there until a female bidan from a neighboring hamlet moved in. Women prefer to call on Mak Da, but when she is unavailable, or when flooding during the mon-soon makes it difficult to reach her house, they are glad to fall back on Pak Su Zali's services.

[111]

Five of the six active bidan kampung were registered by the government as "Untrained Midwives" and presented with a badge and certificate. The sixth, a woman in her seventies, was considered too old. Although the Midwives Act of 1966 states that "all kampung bidans who fail to register before August 1, 1972, must cease to practice midwifery" (Rosina 1975:5), this elderly midwife continued her practice with the knowledge, if not acceptance, of health authorities.

In keeping with the government's policy of utilizing village midwives as motivators of health (Siti Hasmah 1975*b*:5), monthly classes were instituted at the district capital's Health Center in 1976. Previously, bidan kampung had been able to obtain medicines at the government midwife's clinic in Merchang. To induce them to attend classes, these materials were now distributed only at the Health Center at the close of each class. The first class was well attended by bidan kampung who had come from hamlets and villages all over the district. The five registered bidan kampung from Merchang asked me to drive them there and stay for the session.

The staff nurse lectured the village midwives on the importance of advising women about to give birth to their first babies, and those who had given birth previously to eight or more, to deliver in the hospital. Women who have never before given birth, she explained, cannot know whether or not their pelvises are broad enough to allow them to deliver with no problems. Those who have had many children have loose uterine muscles and run a greater risk of postpartum hemorrhage. Women delivering their second to eighth babies should be advised to deliver at home, she said, unless they are carrying twins or have some other unusual condition, since there are not enough beds in the hospital to accommodate ordinary childbirth cases. She told a story of a woman who insisted on delivering her thirteenth child at home and hemorrhaged to death before the ambulance arrived. She stressed the necessity of always calling the government midwife

[112]

when labor begins, because she is the only midwife capable of giving an injection to contract the uterus and control postpartum bleeding.

She described the symptoms of toxemia and advised the village midwives to check their patients regularly for swollen ankles. She asked them to persuade expectant mothers to attend the government midwife's antenatal clinic. She cautioned them never to try to turn a fetus. If there is a short umbilical cord, she said, the cord might tear. If it is done in the early months of pregnancy it can be of no use since the baby turns many times by itself before it is born.

The staff nurse asked if there were any questions, but none were forthcoming. The bidan kampung, outspoken vigorous women in their own communities, were too shy to speak at a public meeting. After the lecture, the staff nurse inspected the bidan's delivery kits and filled their bottles with antiseptic for the perineum and habitane-in-spirit for the umbilical stump.[4] Registered village midwives must supply themselves with a rattan box lined with white cloth, absorbent cotton, string to tie the umbilical cord, scissors to cut it, and cloth to cover the umbilical stump. The staff nurse remarked to me that bidan kampung are independent contractors, not government employees, and therefore it is not the government's responsibility to provide them with supplies.[5]

The staff nurse succeeded in increasing the bidan's awareness of the symptoms of toxemia. Although several had previously mentioned the dangers of toxemia to me, they considered it a rare condition. Attempting to enlist their support for the antenatal clinic, however, was optimistic, considering village ideas of correct behavior. Village Malays are loathe to give advice unless it is specifically requested. Bidan kampung do not oppose the government's antenatal clinic, but they are unlikely to volunteer advice on this or any other matter. It is beyond the realm of possibility that they would advise all primaparas and grand multiparas to deliver at the hospital. Rural Malays consider hospitals places where very sick people go, to be cured with medicines and surgery, or to die. While hospital medicines are valued as augmentations to, or superior versions of, traditional treatments, surgery is not part of the indigenous medical system and is greatly feared. The association of childbirth, a normal and expected event in a woman's life, with surgery and disease seems incongruous to rural Malays. Furthermore, they feel that a woman delivering her first baby is young and ignorant. She, more than any other woman, needs her relatives to comfort her during her travail. Removing her from their protection and subjecting her to the ministrations of strangers in an unfamiliar setting seems to them the epitome of cruelty. Grand multiparas, however, have proved themselves well able to deliver their babies again and again. They need no doctors or nurses to instruct them, or to "cut" them. Although postpartum hemorrhage is justly feared by village Malays, their philosophy of "wait and see if danger arises and then deal with it, since chances are it may never occur," operates in this context as well as in connection with pantang of pregnancy.

Cautioning bidan kampung to stop turning fetuses strikes at the heart of their own antenatal services. One of their primary responsibilities to pregnant clients is to insure that the fetus is positioned head downward throughout pregnancy. Any other position, they feel, will cause backache, stomachache, and leg pains during pregnancy and put the mother and child at risk during labor and delivery.[6]

While the first supervisory session at the Health Center had been very well attended, the next was not. I was unable to drive the bidan that day, and only two went. They had to take the bus, which cost $1.50 for a round trip. Attending the session meant losing a day's pay (about $4.00 for a female rubber tapper). Since they did not feel they were learning anything valuable at the supervisory sessions and there was no increment to their prestige, there was no discernible compensation for them to offset their expenditures. I was not surprised, therefore, to hear from one of the Merchang bidan that very few midwives from other villages had come to the second session. She decided to make that her last time, too.

THE TRAINING OF A BIDAN KAMPUNG

Training of a village midwife begins at an early age. Small daughters and granddaughters often accompany bidan on their rounds. Fatimah brought her four-year-old granddaughter to lenggang perut and *rombak dapur* (the ceremony that ends the postpartum period) as much for the fun of the feast (kenduri) that follows as for the opportunity of showing her the procedures. Sapiah's seven-year-old daughter played hooky from school whenever she had a chance to tag along while her mother examined patients or delivered babies.

Aside from this subliminal education, which she receives throughout her childhood, a prospective midwife's first instruction is in massage techniques, an important component of postpartum care. Before she is permitted to massage a patient, the student has learned the muscle attachments, which movements will do the most good and which may cause harm, by allowing her hands to be manipulated by her teacher and taken through the motions until she can be trusted to do them herself. The student bidan sits on one side of the patient and her teacher sits on the other. Each massages one leg, the student duplicating her teacher's movements under the latter's watchful eye. They proceed to the arms, and make a complete circuit of the patient's body, ending with a massage of the scalp. After the student bidan has completed her side, the teacher goes over it herself if she feels that the student has not yet mastered the technique, since one of the precepts of Malay massage is that both sides must be treated evenly. Then the patient is instructed to turn on her belly. The bidan completes the massage by flexing her patient's knees, cross-

[115]

ing her legs and pressing them against her back.

Under her teacher's hands, the student's hands discover the body parts of the fetus and the signs that will tell her how far a pregnancy has advanced. She watches her teacher "adjust" a misplaced fetus and turn a breach presentation, and places her hands over those of her teacher in order to understand the procedures manually as well as visually. She accompanies her instructress on obstetrical calls and gradually takes over some of the responsibilities. She sits at the feet of the woman in labor, opposite her teacher, and helps massage her legs and abdomen to decrease discomfort. When the patient reaches the last part of the second stage of labor, the student holds her legs in position, knees flexed and legs at a sufficient angle from the body for the midwife to monitor her labor's progress.

Although Chen (1974—1975:341) writes that no vaginal examinations are performed by bidan kampung, and Wylde (1957: 131) and Chen (1974—1975:341) state that the midwife is not permitted to see the baby emerge and conducts the delivery by feel alone, I have not found this to be the case. Deep penetration to ascertain the degree of cervical dilation is not performed, but superficial vaginal examination is frequently done to monitor the baby's passage down the birth canal. It is true that the mother "lies supine and is covered by her sarong as modesty prescribes" (Chen 1974—1975:341), however, from time to time the bidan raises the sarong sufficiently to allow herself (and no one else, unless she is training a student) a clear view of the perineum. After she has satisfied herself, the sarong is once more pulled down. Friends and relatives assembled in the delivery room must sit near the patient's head. From this vantage point it is impossible to see the actual delivery take place. As an apprentice bidan kampung, sitting at the patients' feet, I saw many babies' heads and shoulders slip out of their mothers' bodies.

When I asked the midwives if it had ever been the custom in Trengganu to deliver babies by feel only, or if they had heard of

[116]

midwives in other states of Malaysia who had been limited to this procedure, they laughed and asked me if this was how things were done in America. They had never heard of anything quite so bizarre. A bidan must be courageous, since the danger inherent in viewing birth may cause her to risk her eyesight, but who would be so foolhardy as to attempt to deliver a human life without seeing what was happening?

Since Chen mentions such "blindfold" deliveries taking place in Trengganu (1974–1975:352), one cannot hypothesize that he is referring to some other Malaysian state where such a practice may actually exist. I am convinced that it can never have been widespread, if in fact it ever occurred. "Facts" of this sort, based on hearsay evidence rather than participant observation, not only distort the ethnographic record but can be seized upon by those eager to demonstrate the inadvisability of permitting native practitioners to deal with medical problems.

After the student bidan has learned the art of massage, assisted in a number of births, and helped clean up after deliveries, she is allowed to bathe and dress the newborn. While the student is learning and observing, her teacher is observing her. A bidan must be brave. The responsibility for human lives rests on her. She cannot be squeamish about the sight or smell of blood, or of the feces that are often excreted by the laboring woman. She must be aware of supernatural dangers that can occur during delivery, but she cannot be fearful of them. If a student bidan shows that she is strong, patient, and brave, her teacher knows that she has inherited the angin (talent; character traits) necessary for a good bidan. This heritage is not guaranteed. A woman who springs from a long line of bidan kampung may, herself, lack angin. Those who exhibit the requisite qualities, however, whatever their known parentage, must have inherited them. If a bidan's adopted daughter, or other student whose own mother and grandmother were not bidan, shows angin, her teacher will not ascribe it to her instruction but to an unknown bidan in the

[117]

student's family tree, a many-times-removed grandmother.

The final test of a student bidan is to deliver a baby by herself. By the time she has reached this stage, she has already been instructed in some of the birth ritual. On the whole, obstetrical and nursing expertise precedes ritual expertise, but all are necessary for the performance of the bidan's duties. During pregnancy, her ritual performance is limited to lenggang perut. During labor and delivery there are precautionary measures to be followed, which increase in number if labor is long or difficult.[7] In particularly serious cases most bidan reach the end of their "inner knowledge" and a bomoh must be called in. During the postpartum period, a midwife may be called upon to treat the mother or child for simple cases of lekat kenan, or to release them from the danger of having undergone an abnormal birth, for instance one where the baby's head or shoulders seemed to be stuck in the birth canal,[8] or where the baby was born with the cord looped around its neck. At the close of the puerperium she must *rombak dapur* (dismantle the "roasting bed"), a ceremony that releases the mother and child from the dangers of childbirth and returns them to everyday life. Rombak dapur is important for the bidan, as well as for her patients. If she is not ritually released, her vision may dim from having witnessed a woman's vagina produce life.

When the student bidan has reached a satisfactory level of performance, her teacher tells her that she may *terima* (receive her blessings to practice on her own). She prepares nasi semangat, the invariable accompaniment to all occasions marking a rite of passage. Even if the teacher is her own mother, she must present her with a standardized gift of cloth, money, and betel quid ingredients. Without the receipt of the gift, the transfer of knowledge is incomplete. It is also customary for the student to give her teacher part of the proceeds from her first few professional engagements.

The initiation need not be a public affair, and in fact is often done with few people present besides the teacher and student.

[118]

The new bidan does not, thereafter, advertise her availability and newly won professionalism, but waits for people to call upon her services. Her clientele is built up through recommendations of satisfied patients. Malay patients are not noted for their loyalty to particular indigenous medical practitioners regardless of their ability to effect cures, or assist at deliveries without serious mishap. Although isolated failures may be explained as due to a variety of reasons ranging from countermagic to a lack of harmony between patient and healer, bomoh or bidan with a mounting record of failures will soon find their patients have forsaken them.

Every active village midwife, therefore, has been fully trained and is competent in the eyes of her clientele. Characterizing bidan kampung as untrained is an expression of cultural bias in favor of formal schooling over apprenticeship. It is not an objective description of fact.

ANTENATAL CARE

The village midwife is rarely called upon to act as a ritual specialist during pregnancy. Considered a normal condition that requires few changes in behavior, pregnancy is expected to proceed on a largely uneventful course to its ultimate conclusion. Most women, however, have occasion to seek the bidan's medical services. She can tell them if they are really pregnant or if their menstrual period is merely delayed. She can ascertain how far a pregnancy has advanced. She can relieve stomachache, backache, and aching legs by massaging the mother and adjusting the position of the fetus. Women who have suffered falls or beatings come to the bidan to be reassured that their baby is still healthy and correctly placed within the womb. The seventh and eighth months of pregnancy are considered optimum times for turning the fetus. Before the seventh month, bidan think it can more easily revert to an "unnatural" position. After the eighth month,

[119]

it occupies too much space inside the uterus for the procedure to be safe.

Many more women visit the government midwife's antenatal clinic than the homes of the village midwives, and they visit the clinic with more frequency and regularity (see table 9).

TABLE 9

ANTENATAL VISITS TO THE GOVERNMENT MIDWIFE'S CLINIC
AND TO BIDAN KAMPUNG
(4 kampung survey)

Clinic		*Bidan kampung*	
no. of visits during pregnancy	*% of total patients*	*no. of visits during pregnancy*	*% of total patients*
0	3 (2)	0	26 (18)
1	3 (2)	1	14 (10)
2	9 (6)	2	21 (15)
3	13 (9)	3	27 (19)
4	27 (19)	4	6 (4)
5	14 (10)	5	4 (3)
6	23 (16)	6	1 (1)
7	3 (2)		
8	3 (2)		
10	3 (2)		
N = 70	101%	N = 70	99%
Total visits—313		Total visits—134	

The government midwife tests their blood and urine and measures their weight and blood pressure. Most women were interested in their weight and had heard of *darah tinggi* (literally, high blood, which the indigenous medical system ascribes to "over-

[120]

heated" blood). They willingly gave blood and urine samples but had no clear idea concerning the necessity or significance of the tests.

Informants gave as reasons for attending the clinic:

1. "The government wants us to be healthy, so we should go," and variations on this theme.

2. To corroborate the bidan kampung's diagnosis as to how long a pregnancy had progressed. This estimate was not infrequently at odds with that of the government midwife. In case of disagreement, patients tended to believe the village midwife's pronouncement. The duration of pregnancy is not so pressing a question to women in Merchang as to their American sisters. Deliveries of viable babies were reported to have taken place anywhere from the seventh to the twelfth month. Such late births, which seem to me to belong to the realm of mythology and suggest to American obstetricians a pathological condition that could not possibly result in a live birth, were discussed as rare but perfectly normal occurrences. My assistant's mother, claiming that he was a twelve-month baby, explained that some plants, some animals, and some people take longer to develop than others.

3. Women wanted to be able to call on the government midwife during labor or immediately after delivery, and feared she would not attend those who had not visited her antenatal clinic. Although some preferred not to call her until after the baby was born, they were anxious to receive a shot of ergometrine to ensure uterine contraction and reduce the risk of postpartum hemorrhage. In cases of retained placenta or other dangerous conditions, it was important to have someone present who could summon transportation to the hospital.

4. Several informants claimed that they were forced to go to the antenatal clinic by the government, which would not allow them to get a birth certificate otherwise, effectively keeping the

[121]

child out of school. This, of course, is completely untrue; however, it illustrates the differences in attitudes toward government health services and indigenous medicine on the part of many villagers.

Visits to the bidan kampung were done at the convenience of the mother, and in response to some specific problem or query. Visits to the clinic had to be on the days assigned, did not necessarily correspond to any immediate felt needs on the part of the mothers, and had, to some people, a positive quality of paternalism, and to others, a negative quality of coercion. Both positive and negative qualities perceived by the village women entail some suspension of independent volition. This is at odds with the workings of the indigenous medical system. Indigenous practitioners come only when called, rarely give advice unless specifically requested to do so, cannot coerce behavior, and are not expected to feel anger or chagrin if a patient ignores their advice or seeks a second opinion. The popularity of the antenatal clinic proves that this is not an insurmountable problem. Pregnant women visited the government midwife almost three times as often as they did the traditional midwives. In no case, however, did their reasons for attending the clinic include referral from indigenous medical practitioners.

It is interesting that Merchang bomoh are beginning to advise some patients to go to the hospital, and to consult doctors for their ailments. Although the medical establishment sees bomoh as competitors, many of them feel that their services are complementary rather than competitive. One old bomoh, encountering the hospital's health care system for the first time, remarked to me that doctors may be better at curing diseases of the body, but only bomoh can cure sicknesses of the heart and soul. Certain types of indigenous specialists are preferred to doctors because they offer alternate forms of therapy. One example is the *mudin*, specializing in fractures and sprains, whose methods are claimed to work faster and preserve muscles from atrophying, since they do not require casts. Other indigenous specialists have a reputation for healing stubborn cases that have not yielded to orthodox treatments, as for example, a female bomoh renowned for curing fertility problems and dysmenorrhea. Although prophets have been predicting the bomoh's imminent demise for the better part of a century (see Maxwell 1907:306), their ability to fill the interstices left by hospital-based medicine as it is now practiced in rural Malaysia, as well as their practice of magic, assures their continuing viability.

The bidan kampung, although they feel perfectly competent to deal with all but the rarest and most life-threatening emergencies, are in a much more vulnerable position, since their obstetric expertise is duplicated by the competing medical system and their practice is regulated by licensing procedures. On the more traditional east coast, the village bidan is highly respected, and many women still prefer her services to those of the government midwife. In some villages on the west coast, however, where government midwives have been available for decades, traditional midwives perform no deliveries. Their duties are now limited to laundry, cooking, cleaning, bathing the baby, and massaging the mother (McArthur 1962:24). Stripped of her obstetric role and reduced to the status of household help, the traditional bidan's calling will no longer ring so loudly in the ears of village girls.

· 6 ·

Giving Birth in a Malay Village

Practical obstetrical and nursing expertise, in the training of a bidan kampung, take precedence over "inner knowledge." Patients often employ the village midwife, during their pregnancies, in her capacity as medical advisor and masseuse and rarely call upon her to act in her role as adept of the supernatural. Childbirth in Merchang, however, is not only a physiological event necessitating medical care, but a stage in a rite of passage as well, requiring spiritual prophylaxis and ritual expertise. A competent midwife knows how to ease her charge's way into the world and protect the vulnerable mother and child from attacks by envious spirits.

It was the curiosity of the archangel Gabriel that created these spirits. God entrusted the Breath of Life into Gabriel's hands and ordered him to place it near Adam's nostrils so that his still lifeless body might be animated. Gabriel opened his hands before reaching his destination, and the Breath of Life escaped. Having no body to receive it, the Breath became hantu, the disembodied older siblings of humankind. Like all siblings, hantu are sometimes beset with feelings of envy toward their younger brothers, the children of Adam, since humans are beings of the light while spirits must live forever in darkness. And like human siblings, they occasionally find ways to even the score.

[124]

Hantu, I was told, are like dogs. If left to their own devices, they will rarely attack. Unlike dogs, however, they are invisible. One therefore runs the risk of inadvertently disturbing them, stepping on their houses, or urinating and defecating in their territory. In such cases they may prove to be vindictive, but they are never truly vicious unless they are harbored by people who use them to harm others. These practitioners of black magic make a compact for the mutual benefit of sorcerer and spirit. If their "master" neglects them or dies, leaving them unfed and uncared for, spirits may turn feral and inflict injury and even death upon their "master's" neighbors.

The most feared spirits on the east coast are the *Hantu Raya* (Mighty Spirits), a royal family whose power is great but whose range is limited. Each is rajah of his own territory and does not travel far beyond the confines of his parish. When my neighbor's first baby was born dead after three days of labor, its death was widely attributed to the Hantu Raya. The spirit, people said, was not acting on its own initiative but at the behest of a powerful bomoh who had a grudge against the baby's father. Several years before his marriage, he had fallen in love with the bomoh's daughter-in-law. He suggested that she provoke her husband into divorcing her so she could then marry him. She refused his offer and repeated the story to her father-in-law, who swore vengeance. All signs pointed to the Hantu Raya: the baby's little corpse was bruised along its entire length by the hantu's spectral pinches. The mother would have died too, but her family wisely removed her to an inland village thirty miles away, far enough from the local Hantu Raya's territory to allow her to recover from her ordeal.

Women in childbirth must be protected from the Spirits of the Earth (Jin Tanah, the earth genie, and Jin Hitam, the black genie), who are attracted by the sweet blood of parturition dripping through the floorboards to the ground below. The "dirty" blood of menstruation does not appeal to hantu, and small

[125]

amounts of blood from wounds are beneath their notice, but a great deal of blood lost by a woman whose labors have already depleted her semangat may prove irresistible.

Dangers may arise from beings who are classified as hantu but have human origins. Few reports on Malay childbirth fail to mention the dreadful *penanggalan* and *langsuir* or *pontianak* (McHugh 1959:79; Skeat 1972 passim; Winstedt 1951:22; Colson 1971:65; Chen 1973:199–200; Chen 1974–1975:338). The langsuir or pontianak (she is known by one or the other of these names in many states of Malaysia) is a vampirelike creature who was once an ordinary woman. She takes on demonic form after dying in childbirth. According to some accounts (McHugh 1959:79) she is strangely deformed. Not only has her behavior reversed itself from nourishing babies to destroying them but her body has undergone a reversal as well. Her breasts, the organs of nourishment, have left their normal position and are now located on her back. Under them is a cavity through which she sucks the blood of newborn babies. According to others (Skeat 1972:326), she is a beautiful seductive woman who can easily tempt an unsuspecting man into marrying her. Her face is lovely, but her long black hair conceals the horrible hole. A clever man can change a langsuir into a human woman if he places a nail or other long, hard, pointed piece of iron or steel into the hole. After its insertion, the gap closes up, leaving no mark to reveal the langsuir's nature.

The penanggalan could never pretend to be other than what she is: a disembodied woman's head with trailing intestines. One account of her origins says that she studied magic with a devil who taught her how to loosen her head and neck from her body, allowing her to fly about the countryside, seeking women in childbed (Abdullah 1969:115–117). Another (Skeat 1972:327–328) tells of a woman who sat naked in a vat of palm wine to mortify her body as a means of obtaining magical power—singularly outré behavior among people whose modesty dictates that they bathe dressed in a sarong. When a man came upon her unexpectedly, she was so startled that, on trying to escape, she kicked her chin with such force that the skin split around her neck, and her head, with intestines pendant, separated from her body and flew off.

We have previously noted what far-reaching consequences are attributed to the startle reaction. It may deplete one's vital spirit, leaving one open to spirit attacks. A woman startled in pregnancy may pass on the characteristics of the object of her fear to her unborn child. In this legend of the penanggalan, the woman is startled because she has been caught attempting to gain control over unseen forces in a socially disapproved manner. Rather than losing any part of her own spirit, she herself joins the spirit world.

One of my Malay friends from a west coast state told me yet another story of the penanggalan. She was originally a flirtatious woman. One day, as she was leaning out of the window of her house, smiling and calling to passing men, her husband caught her and grabbed hold of her body to pull her back into the house. In the struggle her head came loose from her body, together with her intestines, leaving her husband with an empty shell while she went flying away.

Both of these birth demons, the langsuir and the penanggalan, were women who reversed, or did not fulfill, their normal roles. The langsuir was unsuccessful in completing her womanly task of giving birth. She is an empty woman, whose gaping hole is dangerous and threatening. She can only be controlled by the introduction of a phallic object into her yawning pit. She is restored to humanity by the power of this symbolic sex act. The penanggalan's openly immodest behavior has already put her in opposition to the ideal of Malay womanhood, the deferential, compliant, and circumspect wife. It takes just another small turn in the world of myth for her to lose not only her womanliness but her humanity as well.

In many parts of Malaysia these demons are forces to be reckoned with today rather than figures from a long-dead cultural nightmare. My young language teacher in Kuala Lumpur, a native of Perak who was urbanized to the point of wearing short skirts, told me that a friend of her mother's had been married to a pontianak. She appeared on the beach for three successive days, beckoning to him. She was far lovelier than any woman of his kampung. He knew she was a pontianak because of the hole in her back, but she was too attractive for him to resist. On the third day he came prepared with a nail to effect her transformation. They married and she soon became pregnant. After the child was born, she remembered her grisly origins, ate up the baby, and disappeared forever.

The *bajang*, a spirit with nonhuman origins, is a problem for women in some states of Malaysia. Colson describes her as a female hantu who eats fetuses and drinks the milk of lactating women. He also mentions a *hantu kopek*, who departs from his description of the bajang only insofar as she sports long and pendulous breasts (Colson 1971:63−64). Chen (1974−1975: 339−340, 1975:105) writes that the striations of pregnancy are thought to be the scars that result from the bajang's attacks. These spirits are not feared as birth demons in present-day Kelantan or Trengganu. There is a hantu named Sang Kopek, but she is invoked only on occasions when it is necessary to invite all known hantu by name to a feast or celebration, for fear of angering an uninvited spirit. None of the local hantu is called bajang, though several, possibly through the workings of folk etymology, are known as bujang (unmarried person). Among the hantu who must be remembered on certain ceremonial occasions are Mak Bujang Hitam (The Unmarried Black Mother), the companion of the Tiger Spirit, and Bujang Tujuh, Janda Sembilan (The Seven Old Maids and the Nine Widows or Divorcees), some of whose names are the Moldy Old Maid (Bujang Lapuk), the Old Maid Who Cannot Control Her Urination (Bujang Beser) and Miss Fever Unabating (Mek Demam Tak Kebah). The possessors of these charming names, while they are fully capable

[128]

of bringing sickness to their human victims, do not specialize in obstetrical problems. Women in Merchang do not attribute striations of pregnancy to spirit attacks. Most of them believe they are due to the pregnant woman's scratching her own abdomen, and several added they could also be caused by stretching of the skin as the fetus grows.

Although the langsuir was known in Trengganu in the past, she was not mentioned as one of the dangers of childbirth by any of my informants. Upon further questioning, one of the oldest bomoh told me that in the past langsuir had been a problem, but people now knew how to deal with them. There had not been any trouble for as long as he could remember. He advocated piercing the demon's neck with iron or steel while repeating the appropriate spell.[1]

Iron and steel are used for defense against inimical supernatural influences throughout pregnancy and childbirth in Merchang. During the lenggang perut, the bidan touches a razor blade to the skin of the mother-to-be, both as a deterrent to spirits and an instrument to harden her semangat. Kelantanese people include a sharp piece of steel in the materials buried with the afterbirth, the baby's older sibling who resembles the older siblings of mankind, the hantu. After the umbilical cord is cut, the baby is protected against the onslaughts of hantu, and his newly acquired semangat is strengthened, by the knife or scissors held by the aunt or grandmother who cradles him. This dual protection is continued throughout the neonatal period. Sharp metal objects are placed above or below the baby's cradle, and other sharp objects from the plant and animal world may be added to the collection. Rice and iron, the symbols of Man's control of the universe, are the two major Malay material defenses against encroachment from the forces of chaos beyond human control.

Sharp and spiny pineapple plants or screwpine are placed under the houses of women in labor throughout Malaysia. On the west coast they serve as thorny traps for the trailing intestines of

[129]

the penanggalan. East coast women, who do not fear (and in most cases have never heard of) the penanggalan, employ the spiny plants as a protection against the Earth Spirits. While thorns are almost always utilized at some point during childbirth, people were not overly concerned about their absence during labor. It was not uncommon for me to find, upon arrival at the home of a woman in labor, that her family had neglected to gather thorny plants. They usually remedied this after the baby's birth on the theory that this, at least, would deter hantu from giving the new mother nightmares. Bidan said that spiky plants were good but not absolutely essential to the mother's well-being. The best protection against hantu is the procedure that the bidan kampung follows soon after arriving at a patient's home.

Before her arrival, the family prepares a mixture of raw rice, salt, diced turmeric, and *asam* (either *Tamarindus indica* or *Garcinia atroviridis* will do), to which one bidan adds soot. The midwife throws this mixture to the four cardinal points of the compass and sprinkles it through the floorboards, reciting an incantation:

> In the name of God the loving and merciful.
> Genie of the Earth, Earth Spirit, I surely know your source.
> Hey, I will plant the yellow dove
> The yellow dove will I plant, I alone.[2]
> Become flies![3]
> Hey, I know the reason for your origins.
> Listen well to my commands,
> For if you do not, I swear I will curse you.
> Fly away, become dust, become wind.
> My teacher has taught me to be effective.
> My teacher is effective through the holy words
> There is no God but Allah and Muhammad is His Prophet.
> Speak and say that God is One.
> To Him do we pray.
> He neither gives birth nor was He born,
> And there is none like him.[4]

Each of the ingredients contains properties that make the mixture antithetical to the spirit world. Rice, a component of all

Malay magical procedures to keep hantu at bay, provides the elemental qualities of earth and water to balance the air and fire of the spirits. A bidan who added soot said that its blackness added to the mixture's efficacy since black is the color of the earth spirits. Turmeric and asam's royal yellow colors remind the spirits that the woman in labor is under the protection of the sultan of Trengganu whose purported ancestor, King Solomon, vanquished the genies.

Salt is used in two other Malay birth rituals: the preparation of the afterbirth for burial and the "opening of the mouth" of the newborn. The bidan's reasons for using salt in the protective mixture she strews during labor combine the reasons for its use on the other two occasions. The word describing salt's saline quality, *masin*, is also used to describe effective speech. Using it to "open the newborn's mouth" aids him in developing into a persuasive conversationalist. Using it as an accompaniment to the bidan's spell adds to the effectiveness of her words. The afterbirth is sprinkled with salt since it shares some of the hantu's characteristics. It is the infant's sibling, just as the hantu are humanity's sibs. Like the hantu, it lacks some basic human characteristics (although its lack is the opposite of the hantu's because the afterbirth has no heat or air to animate its flesh, while the spirits have no flesh to enclose their heat and air), and envies its more complete human brothers and sisters. Salt is a durable material, immune from decay itself and a preservative of other substances. Its use as *materia magica* has a wide distribution.[5]

Salt appears to be another mechanism, together with iron and rice, to keep spirits where they belong, a constant theme of Malay spells. Human spirits must be strengthened in their hour of danger and protected against inadvertently leaving the body, and hantu must be persuaded to stay within their own domain, lest they destroy the balance of the universe and harmony within the bodies of humans, by crossing the boundaries that separate the material from the immaterial. Although most women accomplish the birth of their children without undergoing anything more

serious than a certain amount of productive discomfort, childbirth is, nevertheless, potentially fraught with the utmost danger
to both mother and child. Gatekeeping mechanisms for keeping
the world of the hantu and the world of humanity separate are
essential for the protection of the couple.

Supernatural presences are not all to be feared. Sometimes
beneficent beings come to the aid of women in childbirth. They
are the Seven Celestial Midwives, the *bidandari*, who are regularly
invoked by bidan kampung at the ceremony that releases the
mother and child from the postpartum period. Their name has
had an interesting evolution since its Sanskrit beginnings. The
original word, bidadari, refers to the beautiful nymphs of Indra's
paradise, the heavenly dancing girls. Addition of the letter *n* has
brought the word closer to the world of the rural Malay, and its
meaning has changed to fit the remade name. The Indian temp-
tresses have become heavenly bidan kampung concerned with
the welfare of women in childbirth. A woman in her last extrem-
ity, deserted by mortal helpers, may be delivered by these heavenly midwives. My closest neighbor, Noh, told me that her own
birth was attended by bidandari. Her mother, in labor for seven
days, was all alone. Her husband was at work and the bidan
kampung had gone home. Suddenly seven beautiful smiling
ladies descended from the sky. They eased her pain, delivered
her baby, and washed the mother and child. When they had
finished, they ascended once more to *kayangan* (etymologically
Siva's heaven, distinct from *syurga*, the Muslim heaven). The
neighbors, surprised to hear a baby crying, came in to find the
mother clean and comfortable and the infant washed and swaddled. This auspicious beginning has left Noh with the ability to
see angels, who have visited her home several times. Her spiritual
capabilities were recognized by her father-in-law, an important
bomoh, who offered to teach her after refusing instruction to his
son. She, however, declined, fearing marital discord as much as
she feared dealings with the spirits.

[132]

Giving Birth in a Malay Village

Childbirth poses a particular problem to women of royal blood. A surprising number of villagers, including some of the poorest, claim descent from royalty. They express their nobility in no way other than the preparation for the birth of their children. A bidan must attach a royal yellow cloth to the four walls above such a woman's head and place an open umbrella, the symbol of her rank, upon the outstretched cloth. If these measures are not taken, the denial of her royal heritage might increase the difficulty of her labor.

Although the outcome of most labors is expected to be a normal healthy baby, Malay folklore abounds in stories of unnatural births. I was often told "true" stories of women giving birth to snakes, monitor lizards, butterflies, and eggs. There may be factual evidence in support of "egg" births. For reasons unclear to medical science, the incidence of molar pregnancies, about 1:1,000 gestations in the United States, increases to 1:200 in Asian countries (Holvey and Talbott 1972:818). The hydatidiform mole is the end stage of a degenerating pregnancy in which the entire placenta is transformed into a large number of edematous vesicles which are usually described as resembling a bunch of grapes, but can with equal justification be compared to a clutch of birds' eggs. Considering the relatively high incidence of molar pregnancies among the Malay population, there is a good likelihood that such a delivery has been observed by bidan kampung who interpreted the event in the light of beliefs about unnatural births. This tangible evidence of a woman's having given birth to something other than a human child lends credence to accounts of other unusual births for which such evidence cannot be marshaled.

Unnatural births, other than egg deliveries, usually are the twins of normal births. The snakes, lizards, and butterflies of obstetrical myth accompany their human siblings into the world and, for the rest of his or her life, live near the human twin as a benevolent presence dimly glimpsed from time to time. The

[133]

bidan and bomoh of Merchang consider it impossible to change the form of these unusual offspring. Tok Hitam, a famous female bomoh from Kuala Dungun, however, claimed to know a method of changing "eggs" into a human child. One must place seven cloths, each of a different color, into a container. These cloths, she explained, were like those used in lenggang perut. You must add thread of seven colors, *tepung tawar* (the neutralizing rice paste used in Malay magic), and raw rice that has been steeped in water. The container is then ready for the "eggs." The final step is the addition of *air tawar*—magically treated "neutralizing" water, prepared by the recitation of the following incantation over a pail of water:

> Nahun naham, I want to end the shuddering fear,
> A bit of sweat, accursed heat.
> My labors will make your standing illusion fall.
> May your badi leave and mine take its place.
> May your jinggi leave and mine take its place.
> May your power leave and mine take its place.
> I stand alongside Allah with the holy words
> There is no God but Allah
> And Muhammad is His Prophet.

The illusion referred to in the spell is the appearance of the "eggs." Tok Hitam explained that the woman actually gives birth to a human child, which only seems to look like "eggs." Her magic can take away the illusion and present the true form of the child to view. She never had a chance to prove the value of her treatment since whenever the opportunity arose and she hurried over to assist the stricken family, she found, to her anger, that they had already buried the "eggs."[6]

The next time the subject of unusual births arose in Merchang, I mentioned Tok Hitam's claims to Sapiah. She said that while she had often heard of women giving birth to "eggs," she had never heard of any method for changing them into a human baby and would not believe it possible unless she saw it with her own eyes.

A DIRECTIONAL SYSTEM FOR GIVING BIRTH

Accounts of Malay childbirth by English writers (Skeat 1972: 333; Winstedt 1920:86, 1951:105; Wilkinson 1957:41) describe how the bidan or bomoh chooses a lucky place for the infant's birth by repeatedly dropping a hatchet blade into the ground below the house until the blade sticks upright in the earth. Chen (1974−1975:340; 1975:105) does not mention any method for finding a lucky place, but does state that "the woman [is] always made to lie parallel to the main irrigation canal or stream that is nearest the village, with her feet pointing down-stream so as to symbolically facilitate childbirth."

In Merchang, neither the bidan nor the bomoh used a hatchet to choose an auspicious place nor was the parturient woman's body aligned with any body of water. The midwife's method of facilitating childbirth is one that might easily be overlooked or mistaken for an adjustment undertaken for the woman's comfort or the midwife's convenience. About half an hour before the first delivery I observed, the bidan asked the mother to move slightly to the left. After the event, I asked the bidan, among other questions, why she had wanted the mother to shift her position. She answered that the mother had not been in the proper position to give birth on Monday. It emerged, after many discussions with midwives and healers, that bomoh in Trengganu have a daily directional system reminiscent of those described by Skeat (1972:558) which should be followed by those embarking on some serious undertaking, or a long or dangerous trip, and that bidan use similar systems to guide their patients through childbirth.

The first system I charted, with Sapiah's assistance (fig. 1), uses each direction for an entire day and does not show the days following one another in any obvious order. I was not able to arrive at a coherent rationale for the association of days and directions since neither she nor any other bidan in Merchang was aware of any underlying theory. They used the method unques-

[135]

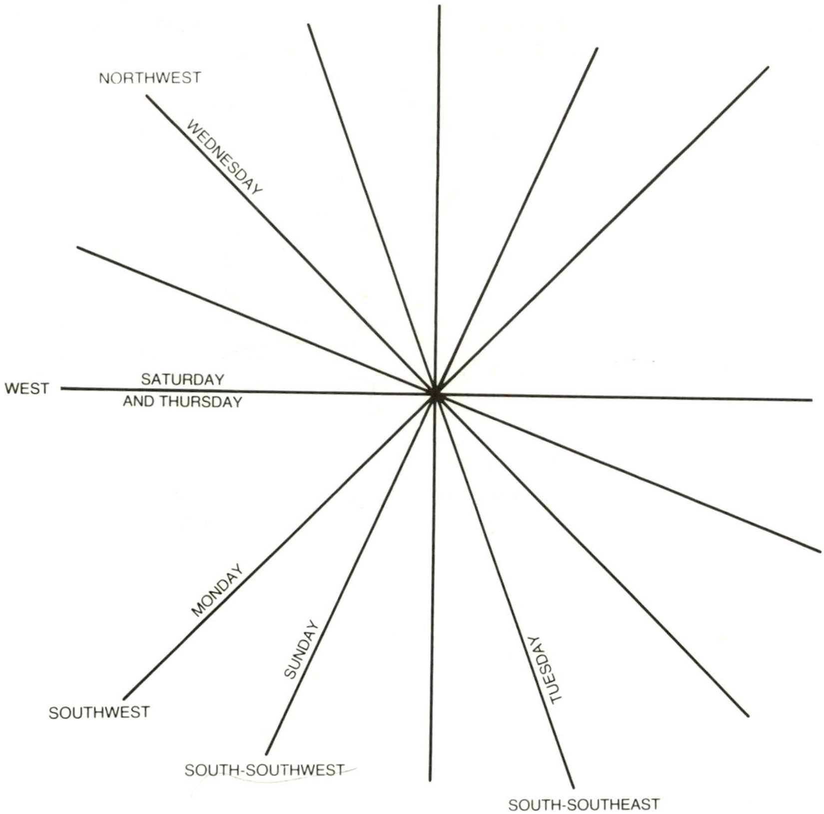

NORTHWEST

WEDNESDAY

WEST

SATURDAY
AND THURSDAY

MONDAY

SUNDAY

TUESDAY

SOUTHWEST

SOUTH-SOUTHWEST

SOUTH-SOUTHEAST

Figure 1. Sapiah's Directional System for Childbirth

tioningly as part of the "inner knowledge" they had learned from their teachers. The Malay student is not encouraged to ask questions. It is only the exceptional individual who ponders the meanings of the knowledge he or she has been taught. Tok Hitam, a bomoh and former bidan of wide learning and venerable age (she claimed to be over 100 years old), was such a person. In her directional system (fig. 2), the days follow one another in counter-

[136]

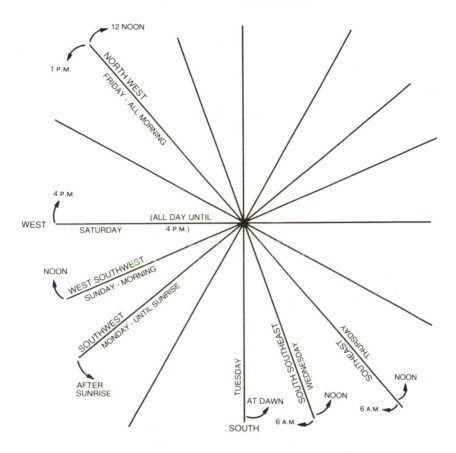

Figure 2. Tok Hitam's Directional System for Childbirth

clockwise sequence, and there are slight adjustments for different
times of day. Each day is associated with a prevailing wind. Both
days and winds have intrinsic measures of "heat" corresponding
to humoral, rather than thermal, measurements. When the heat
of the day matches the heat of the direction, the undertaking will
be lucky and birth will be easy. Starting with the "hottest" and

[137]

proceeding to the "coldest," the days of the week and directions of the compass are given below:

HOT

Direction	Day
1. Northwest (*barat laut*)	Friday
2. South southwest (*selatan raya*)	Saturday
3. South (*selatan*)	Sunday
4. West (*barat*)	Wednesday
5. South southeast (*selatan daya*)	Thursday
6. Southwest (*barat daya*)	Monday
7. West southwest (*barat muda*)	Tuesday

COLD

Using the values of Tok Hitam's chart, we note that in her directional system the days that match their directions in "heat" are Friday, Monday, and Thursday. They are the easiest days on which to give birth. Somewhat harder is Tuesday, which is one step "colder" than its corresponding direction, followed by Wednesday, two steps colder than the prevailing winds of its direction. Harder still is Saturday, two steps hotter than its direction, and hardest of all is Sunday, five steps hotter than its corresponding compass point. According to this system, the larger the discrepancy in intrinsic heat, the greater the difficulty.

In both systems the possible positions cluster around south and west. Easterly and northerly directions are avoided. North is associated with death—corpses are buried with their heads pointing north. People try to avoid sleeping with their heads facing in this direction. A woman who attempts to give birth facing north is actively courting danger. The east is avoided because it is the opposite of west, the holy direction toward Mecca, which Malays face when they pray.[7] Since east is opposite to the holy direction, it carries implications of abandonment by Heaven, leaving the way open for satanic influences.[8]

[138]

Friday, the Islamic sabbath, is also the "hottest" day of the week. Bomoh do not ordinarily practice on Friday. Their treatment is said to be ineffective from sunset to sunset on the holy day. Traditional herbal remedies are most effective when they have been gathered on Tuesday, the day farthest from the sabbath and the "coldest" according to this system. It is also the day on which student bomoh are examined by their teachers and, if they prove to have learned their lessons well, are permitted to present the teacher with ritual gifts and receive his approval to practice their art. The distance of the Islamic sabbath from the day sacred to the activities of the bomoh, both in its temporal position in the week's round and in its symbolic position of relative intrinsic heat, points up the conflict between Islamic orthodoxy and Malay folk beliefs, a conflict that is consciously perceived by indigenous healers as well as by Islamic authorities. It is, perhaps, not an accident that the least congruent day for childbirth is Sunday, the Christian sabbath.

Bidan recognize another system based on the four elements. The first day of each lunar month corresponds to earth, the second to air, the third to fire, the fourth to water, and the fifth begins the cycle anew. Since earth and water are cold elements, when they are in the ascendancy labor will tend to be long and delivery slow. On days when air and fire are in the ascendancy, these hot elements will hasten labor and speed delivery. This system is based on the principle that coolness is conducive to a baby's development in the womb while heat drives it out. Since this system is fixed and cannot be manipulated, it is part of the midwife's theoretical background but not part of her technique. Directional systems, however, were employed by village midwives for every birth at which I was present. On each occasion the direction in which a laboring woman was advised to face (as shown on my compass) was the proper direction for that day according to one or the other directional system. Women were rarely asked to move into the proper position until it was clearly indicated to the bidan (if not to others present) that birth would ake place. After the baby's birth, the bidan would often turn to me and remark on the effectiveness of her system.

The Malay midwife, like the native American rain dancer, chooses the time for her rituals wisely. The rain dancer waits for a time when rain is a distinct possibility which may be helped along by human efforts. He does not waste his ritual by performing it in the middle of a regularly recurring drought season. The Malay bidan, too, saves her "inner knowledge" for a time when the probability of obtaining the desired effect is high. She does not claim that her system is indispensable; she does not say that without it the child would be born sick or deformed. She merely uses it to encourage the infant to arrive more swiftly and with less difficulty than it would if the system were not employed.

THE BOMOH'S ROLE DURING CHILDBIRTH

As a general rule, the bomoh is not called upon to assist a woman in labor unless the midwife feels that the case has gone beyond her capabilities as sole practitioner. The bomoh who assist at difficult births have access to different, and sometimes more sophisticated, treatments than the bidan, but their methods are no more coercive. One bomoh calls the baby's semangat with the same sound Malays use to call their chickens (kurrrr).[9] Where the semangat goes the body must follow, and so the baby is encouraged to make its way into the world. But just as a chicken may or may not respond to its owner's call, so may the baby respond, or not, to the charm, which does not compel behavior. Another bomoh said that a baby is like a fruit. When it is ripe it will be born, and there is no use reciting spells or performing rituals with the intention of hastening its untimely arrival. His jampi,[10] presented below, is meant to enhance the safety of the mother and child, and to keep the mother's mind on holy matters instead of on her pain. All of the interpretations of this incantation were derived from conversations with the bomoh who recited it.

Giving Birth in a Malay Village

In the name of God. First of all I want to put a secret in its proper place. I, the physician, had not yet been born. The Light had not yet emerged from the Darkness. During that time, the Light was manifest within the Lord. The earth and sky had not yet separated. The Heavenly Throne was not yet erected. The Book of Fate had not yet been written, had not yet been revealed. Heaven and Hell were unknown in that time.

I, the physician, ask that skill be added to luck as it was first decreed. I ask to be inspired to become a physician and a healer, and I utter praises to the Lord.

When the Light of Faith had just begun, when the Divine Pen had begun to inscribe all that was written in the Book of Faith into the Hadith, explaining Heaven and Earth, then came three Utterances. The first Utterance became iron, the second Utterance became the Breath of Life, the third Utterance became semen. The semen swelled and glistened like a white sail and became foam. The foam remained in the Sea of God's Man for an immensely long time, for 70,000 years.

First it was the Sea of Practice, second the Sea of Experience, third the Sea of Thought, fourth the Sea of Reason, fifth the Sea of Coitus, sixth the Sea of Tiredness, seventh the Sea of Patience, eighth the Sea of Foam. The foam was carried by the wind, tossed by the waves, by the seven rolling waves, by the groundswell. Where will the foam land? The foam lands on the banks of Desire where the young casuarina tree grows in the golden land in the kingdom of Rajah Bali Stream of Desire.

Then, the Angel Gabriel descended, took up the foam, and presented himself to the Light of Muhammad. He brought it before the Light of Muhammad. Then, Gabriel himself asked the Light of Muhammad, "My Lord, what is within this foam? Its color is fine, of four kinds and seven colors." Then, Muhammad said, "Oh, Gabriel, if you want to known what is within this foam, fetch the strongest Persian steel. Divide the foam in two, break it in four, shred it in five." Then, Gabriel fetched the strongest Persian steel, divided the foam in two, broke it in four, shredded it in five. Within was revealed a couple. The husband was called the First Haji. The wife was called Lady White Dressed in Flowers. You are truly the first seed of life, the original wind of desire.

Then, Gabriel himself carried it within his own hands for forty days. Its name was Light of Command. Then, Gabriel himself thrust it into the

[141]

father's brain for forty days. Its name was Light of Allah. It fell to his eyes, Light of Lights. It fell to his chest, True Sultan, happy center of the world. It fell to his big toe, King Phallus is his name.

Then it is that you, my lord, must pray, my lord, forty times a day forty times a night. Then it is that you fall to the father's womb for forty days. Di, wadi, mani, manikam. From di comes earth, from wadi comes water, from mani comes fire, from manikam comes air.

Then you fall into your mother's womb, in your mother's womb nine months, ten days. The first month you are called Dot. The second month Light of Beginning. The third month Light of the Soul. The fourth month Light of the Countenance. The fifth month Light of the Womb. The sixth month Abdullah the Slow. The seventh month bow to the right, bow to the left. Bow to the right, you are a son. Bow to the left, you are a daughter. The eighth month Light of Birth. The ninth month your outline and measure can be seen. The tenth, out you come.

You carry the twenty attributes of Muhammad. You know your mother's body. You open your eyes and utter three prayers. The first utterance lifts the soul to the breast. The second utterance the Breath of Life to the breast. The third utterance lifts the vital force. May all your feelings be good. You let yourself breath in the five vital forces as you wave your arms thrice. You have a compass within you from the day you first stand within the magic pentacle and the group of letters alif, lam, Za, ruh, lullah. You call upon your friends Gabriel, Michael, Israfel, Israel, Ali, Omar, Osman, Abu Bakar, Kiraman Katibin.

This jampi is a myth that links the creation of the universe to the birth of the baby for whom the incantation is recited. It begins before the universe had taken form, before life had begun. Even in that primordial time the Light of Muhammad existed, making him first among prophets in his spiritual body as well as last in his physical body. The jampi validates Islam as the first among religions, since even before the creation of the world the judgments of the Book of Fate had been inscribed in the Hadith.[11]

Seventy thousand years, the time that elapsed from the first moment of creation to the beginning of mankind, represents the vastness of God's time, the week of creation expressed in human terms. Seven is a significant number in Malay magic and mythology, particularly in the context of childbirth. The Celestial Midwives number seven; seven sarongs are needed for lenggang perut and for changing "eggs" into human form (a procedure that also employs threads of seven colors). The lepas which carries people over the threshold, from danger to safety, ends with the recitation, "One, two, three, four, five, six, seven, you are released!"

The language of jampi employs multiple meanings for the universe without and the world within Man. The sea may refer to the mythical Sea of Creation, the actual South China Sea, the human bloodstream, or to all simultaneously. The Heavenly Throne is also the heart of humanity, the place where God is enthroned. The wind and the waves are not only part of the mythic representation of the Great Sea of Creation, but refer as well to the wind of desire and waves of excitement within the human breast. The golden country is the woman's body; the casuarina trees, whose foliage resembles pubic hair, symbolize the female external genitalia. When the foam (semen) reaches the golden country, the first human couple is created. Within the foam, like a double homunculus, is the ideal Malay man and wife. The husband is a haji who has made his pilgrimage to Mecca, and his wife is the White Flower, symbol of purity. The couple represents the mortal and his immortal soul, as well as the first human pair.

The jampi ends by recounting the creation of the yet unborn child for whom the bomoh recites his spell. It traces the child's development from its earliest beginnings within its father's brain through all the stages of gestation. First it is a speck, so small it cannot be seen. In the second month it has just begun to form. By the third month it has received its soul. Many rural Malays feel that before the third month performing an abortion does not

[143]

incur the sin of murder. After the third month, deliberate termi-
nation of a pregnancy would mean destroying a human soul.
During the fourth and fifth months the fetus takes on human
shape. By the seventh month a midwife can ascertain the baby's
sex by noting whether it is located primarily on the left or right
side of its mother's womb.[12] The right side, associated with purity
and rationality, is the side on which the male baby develops; the
left, reserved for dirty tasks connected with our animal nature, is
the female's side.

The baby's twenty characteristics are the outward signs of
humanity, the *sifat*, contrasted in mystical writings with the *zat*,
the hidden esoteric aspects or true essence. The three prayers
uttered by the newborn endow him with the inward components
of his being. The first, the soul (*ruh*), departs from the body at
death. The second, the breath of life (*nyawa*), is related to the
Greek *pneuma*, both conceptually and etymologically. The newborn must inhale the nyawa within seconds after he is born or his
physical body will not be animated. The third is semangat, the
spirit of life that pervades the universe. The semangat is closely
associated with the body throughout a person's lifetime, but may
be depleted if it is startled or if the body has been weakened by
sickness or overwork. Loss of semangat leaves the body open to
spirit attacks which would not succeed if directed against whole
and healthy people.

The five vital forces and five directions are our senses. The
inner compass refers to the directional systems, to the conscience
that keeps one on the proper path, and to fate, the course that
one's life will take. The letters have multiple meanings as well.
Alif stands for Allah, and lam completes the shorthand for God's
name. Za, ruh and lullah (the last is not a letter but a variant of ila
Allah) stand for Azrael, the angel of death, a reminder of every-
man's mortality, and for *zikir ruh Allah*, which means "the soul
remembers and praises God." The newborn infant calls upon the
four archangels, Gabriel, Michael, Israfel, and Israel, and the

four Companions of the Prophet, Ali, Omar, Osman, and Abu Bakar. Kiraman Katibin are the Recording Angels; one records good deeds and the other evil.

This jampi can be compared with the Cuna Indian birth song, the Mu-Igala, made famous by Lévi-Strauss (1963*a*:186–205). Indeed, their very differences constitute a mythic reversal to gladden the hearts of Structuralists. The Cuna song begins with a long and detailed recounting of events that transpired in the world of ordinary reality. It tells of the midwife's arrival, of her inability to help the laboring mother, of her trip to the shaman's house to request his aid, and of their return to the sick woman's house. It is not until this story has been told at great length that the scene shifts to the realm of the supernatural, the abode of Mu. The laboring woman is sick because Mu, the power that forms the fetus, has captured her soul. The shaman must send his own soul into the spirit world to wrest the sick woman's soul from Mu and her daughters. The battleground is neither in the sky nor in some invisible dimension, but within the pregnant woman's uterus, a world peopled with threatening animals and powerful spirits. Thus, in the Cuna song, the macrocosm has become the microcosm, the unseen universe is contained within a woman's genitals.

In contrast to the prosaic opening of the Cuna song, the Malay incantation begins in the time before Creation, in the vastness of unimaginable space. Nothing exists except God and the Light of Muhammad. The Universe is pregnant with life, and Creation is imminent. As the jampi progresses, the story of Creation narrows to an account of the creation of the first human couple, the primeval ancestors of the very baby whose mother is the audience for the bomoh's chant. The jampi moves further from the general to the particular, from the mythic to the real, as it recounts the stages of the baby's development. It ends with the birth of the baby into the world of familiar human occurrences.

Lévi-Strauss emphasizes the woman's transition from prosaic reality to myth, her reliving of pain through psychological aware-

[145]

ness, and the language, provided by the shaman, for the expression of her otherwise inexpressible psychic state. The representations evoked by the shaman's song, he believes, have the power to modify organic functions; the details of the myth elicit a corresponding organic reaction.

Lévi-Strauss' brilliant exegesis is based upon a text that had passed through many hands. The song was recited by an old shaman to an uninitiated bilingual Cuna Indian who translated it literally into Spanish. The Spanish version was revised by Holmer (Holmer and Wassen 1953) and translated into English. Basing an interpretation upon a text several times removed from its source presents serious problems, since

> Like so many other species of literary composition of a magical or mystical nature, the song of Mu-Igala cannot be rightly understood except by the medicine man himself or by those initiated by him. It is possible to make a thoroughly literal translation of its contents, but its hidden meaning remains secret on many points. [Holmer and Wassen 1953:14]

Lévi-Strauss' reading of the chant has come under criticism from ethnographers who, unlike him, have done fieldwork among the Cuna. The details of the shaman's song, they say, cannot evoke corresponding physiological changes since the words are often incomprehensible to the patient (Sherzer 1974) who may not even be present during their recitation (Chapin 1976).

I tape-recorded the Malay jampi as the bomoh recited it to a young woman in prolonged and painful labor, giving birth to her first child. Later, I read my transcription back to the bomoh to check its accuracy and translated it under his supervision. Although few of the words were incomprehensible in themselves, I could neither have understood the jampi's allusions nor fathomed the multiple meanings often conveyed by one word or phrase, without the bomoh's painstaking explanations. I wondered how much his patient had understood. Had the details of the chant been clear to her; could the specificity of its symbols evoke a specific organic response? When I questioned the new mother, she remembered the bomoh's incantation but did not recall its content. After she listened to my tape she was able to explain the jampi's general outline and rationale, but many of its inner meanings and symbolic allusions escaped her. If the symbols had been effective—and I believe they had—their power lay in their generality and ambiguity rather than their specificity.

While their roles and mythology are dissimilar, the incantations of both Malay bomoh and Cuna shaman provide a rationale for the woman in protracted labor which puts her pains into a meaningful context with a promised satisfactory ending, rather than allow them to be felt as unproductive and chaotic torment. Her experiences have already placed her outside the normal temporal scheme. The first stage of labor, the period from the onset of regular contractions of the uterus until the cervix is fully dilated, seems alternately to take a long time or no time at all. For the woman in labor there is no sense of living through an ordinary sixty minute hour. The second stage, the period from complete dilation of the cervix through the birth of the baby, which normally takes from twenty to fifty minutes, may seem unimaginably long. In the last hour of my own labor, I felt as though I were in the grip of forces beyond my control, rocked by the long waves and groundswell of my contractions, each of which seemed to follow close in the wake of its predecessor. The medicine man, recognizing the woman's time dislocation, provides her with the device of mythic time, a time controlled by a rationality beyond everyday appearance, in which to rally her forces and concentrate her efforts for a successful conclusion to her labor.

The bidan's directional system and the bomoh's jampi are examples of a theme that runs through Malay culture: the concept of sayang or sesuai.[13] We have noted how, if the fetus is sayang within its mother, neither accident nor deliberate inter-

)n will dislodge it. When the child is born, its name must be
ii with its nature or it will be vulnerable to illness. For a cure
: successful, the patient and healer must be sesuai. If a patient
calls upon a second bomoh for treatment, it is not necessarily a
reflection on the skills of the first. The second may be more sesuai
with the patient or his disease.

Sesuai or sayang usually refer to harmony in relations between
people, between a person and the world, or to conditions within
oneself. Their opposite, bisa, is an intensifier that comes from
without and attacks by enhancing preexisting disharmonies. The
bidan's directional system is not meant to coerce the baby to make
its way into the world, it merely makes sure that the mother is in a
position that is sesuai for that particular day of the week and time
of the day. The harmony thus set up between the laboring
mother and the outside world encourages the baby to emerge.
Similarly, the bomoh's jampi is not the battle cry of a hero who
wrests the mother's soul from the forces of darkness. Its function
is to focus the mother's mind on her task and to make conditions
as sesuai as possible for mother and child.

The bomoh's role during childbirth is far different from that of
the Cuna shaman described by Lévi-Strauss. The shaman has the
starring role in the birth drama. The laboring woman lies passive
while the shaman sends his spirit on a perilous quest, to do battle
with spiritual powers for the possession of her captured soul. The
hero-shaman has more in common with the hero-obstetrician
than he does with the bomoh. Both heroes manipulate the
woman's body, the former with myth and symbol, the latter with
tools, drugs, and commands. If the delivery proves successful, it is
the hero-practitioner rather than the victim-patient who is to be
congratulated for a job well done. The Malay bomoh, like the
bidan, assists the parturient woman rather than manipulating
her. He identifies the woman's reproductive powers with universal creativity, using the deliberate ambiguity of symbols, and
gradually focuses upon the drama of birth taking place within a
particular time and space, and involving a particular mother and

[148]

child. The woman retains the principal role; the bomoh merely aids her in the completion of her task.

The symbolic universe I have described works on different aspects of the situation. It makes a problematic social and biological process more familiar and gives it the appearance of regularity and control. It may work psychologically, and may modify physiological and even biochemical processes. Recent studies can provide a framework in which to discuss such possible avenues for the efficacy of the medical-ritual practitioner's treatment.

Naaktgeboren's studies of psychogenic factors in a variety of animal births demonstrate how fear can slow down and even stop uterine contractions (Arms 1975:130−131). For example, rabbits, who normally expel their litters within the space of ten minutes, stopped after the birth of the first of the litter for periods of up to two hours in response to the presence of a stranger (Naaktgeboren himself). When the disturbing presence was removed, the rest of the litter was born within twenty minutes. The prolongation of labor because of fear is associated with a much higher than normal perinatal mortality rate. Studies involving deer, horses, cattle, rats, and dogs have demonstrated similar responses to those noted by Naaktgeboren in rabbits (Newton 1977).

Uterine dysfunction or inertia appears at different phases of labor with a characteristic pattern. In the latent phase (from 0 to 3 cm. of cervical dilatation), the contractions often are intense, regular, painful, and ineffectual. In the active phase (from 4 cm. to full cervical dilatation) the contractions tend to be irregular, mild, and unproductive (Anderson et al. 1974−1975: II, 238). A recent study (Lederman et al. 1978:495) suggests a biochemical pathway for uterine dysfunction. Anxiety levels in laboring women were correlated with their production of epinephrine. The higher the anxiety level, the more epinephrine was produced, resulting in lower uterine contractile activity and longer phase two labors.

The medicine man's incantation, by reducing the laboring

[149]

woman's anxiety, may reduce her epinephrine production. With her fears under control, her uterine inertia may be counteracted and the normal functioning of productive contractions restored.

Biochemical changes in a woman's body late in pregnancy may prepare her to experience labor with a minimum of pain. Levels of endorphins, substances produced in the brain with a shape and effect similar to that of morphine, increase significantly during the last trimester (Akil et al. 1979:1663), peaking during late labor (Czontos et al. 1979; Goland et al. 1981).[14] These endorphins can mask pain, induce euphoria and, possibly, reduce the memory of pain. It has long been known that the administration of pharmacologically inactive substances can result in a wide range of physiological responses and is particularly valuable for the control of pain. The analgesic effect of these placebos is owing to the production of beta endorphins which they trigger in many patients' brains (Li 1978). Besides reducing epinephrine production, the medicine man's treatment may also provide a placebo effect that changes his patient's biochemistry by encouraging her body to produce higher levels of beta endorphins than ordinarily occur in the course of normal labor.

Before the bomoh is consulted, the bidan has tried all the techniques she was taught as a student, or learned in the course of her career. If labor is prolonged, the bidan may give her patient a decoction of "hot" medicines to drink, and rub lime (calcium oxide, an extremely "hot" material) on her abdomen, to make it an uncongenial place for the baby's further occupancy. The midwife may also employ *minyak selusuh* (magically treated coconut oil over which charms have been recited, used to ease childbirth), to massage her patient's abdomen. She may drop some of this oil from her third finger (the *jari manis*, or sweet finger) into a glass of drinking water. The slipperiness of the oil, enhanced by the spell, is intended to ease the baby's path through the birth canal.

If a woman in labor has strayed from her prescribed feminine

[150]

role during her pregnancy, disobeying or attempting to dominate her husband, she may find it hard to deliver her baby. She runs a similar risk if she has been unfaithful to her husband, even in thought. Malays believe that since women are naturally passive and follow their husbands' lead, a woman who reverses her role may have difficulty in carrying out her normal womanly functions. To restore harmony and order in the universe, and return the erring wife to her proper place, the midwife instructs her husband to step over his wife's supine body three times, in a gesture that graphically illustrates which sex must be on top and which must be in danger of being trodden underfoot, however symbolically, to insure reproductive success. If she is suspected of having touched or thought of another man carnally, she may be asked to drink water into which her husband has dipped his penis. Village Malay men do not appear to be enthusiastic practitioners of oral sex. Those with whom my relationship was relaxed enough to allow discussion of this topic were emphatic in their expressions of disgust at the thought of performing such a nauseating act on a woman. They were not adverse to being the recipients of oral sex, however. Women can sometimes be persuaded to practice it upon their husbands, although they, in turn, feel it is somewhat humiliating. When a woman in childbirth drinks the treated water, her husband's dominance is reestablished and her submission to her wifely duties may facilitate delivery by placing her in her proper position as woman and wife.

If the baby's head crowns but seems to be stuck within the passage for an inordinate length of time, the midwife may oil the mother's hair and, lifting some strands above the place where her fontanelle used to be, recite, "If this hair is slippery, you will slip right out; if this hair is not slippery, you will not slip out."[15] The location of the mother's hair is as important as the spell. The fontanelle is a mysterious spot in the baby's skull, soft and vulnerable and pulsing with life. Holding the hair above the mother's former fontanelle is a remembrance of her own birth. Since she

[151]

was successfully born, the sympathetic vibrations set up between mother and child by the spell should assist him into the world.

If the afterbirth is not expelled within a reasonable time after the baby's birth, both government midwife and traditional midwife massage the fundus of the uterus, exerting some pressure. Bidan kampung also lift the abdomen in an effort to free the placenta, which, they believe, may be trapped by a suddenly descending stomach.

If the newborn's airway is full of mucus, preventing the infant from breathing, the government midwife aspirates it with a rubber bulb syringe. The bidan kampung, lacking such conveniences, sucks the mucus from the baby's passages and spits it out.

A BABY IS BORN IN MERCHANG

I have, until now, described customs as a general script for the acting out of gestation and birth—a script learned from numerous observations and conversations. Since all learning is contextually specific, and since the particulars of each sequence of events require people to improvise their actions from the elements of these cultural scripts, I will recount two cases of childbirth to show how this is done. In both cases the patient, not the practitioner, is the protagonist in the drama of birth. Her wishes must be respected; she is the ultimate arbiter of decisions taken during childbirth. For the majority of births, producing a normal infant after an uncomplicated delivery, this preservation of female autonomy, so alien to most deliveries in America, is strongly conducive to the mother's well-being. Responsibility carries certain risks, however, particularly when the person in command does not have all the facts at her disposal. The first case, an uncomplicated birth attended by a village midwife, illustrates the positive aspects of the traditional medical system; the second, a difficult labor attended by both government midwife and bidan kampung, shows its dangers.

[152]

Giving Birth in a Malay Village

Case no. 1: Senani has a son

At about 8 A.M. Sapiah came to my house to tell me that a woman was in labor. She was a cousin of my assistant on her father's side and related to his wife on her mother's. She had given permission to Sapiah to invite me to be present at the delivery of her baby. She and her husband had come from Kuantan (in Pahang, the neighboring state to the south and west) so that she might give birth at her parents' home. She had already borne five children, including a pair of twins who had died in infancy. Senani's oldest child, Liza, a classmate of my son, had been given years ago to her grandparents to raise, since otherwise their house would have been empty of children and they would have been lonely. The doctor in Kuantan advised Senani to give birth in the hospital, but since he did not suspect a twin birth this time she thought it unnecessary. She had also been examined at the Health Center in Marang (the capital of the district which includes Merchang). The doctor at the Health Center told her that she was carrying twins, but Sapiah was convinced it was only one baby. Her opinion, added to that of the Kuantan doctor, strengthened Senani's resolve to deliver at home. She was having very mild contractions at irregular intervals when we arrived. Sapiah felt Senani's feet and said that she would not deliver very soon. She said that if the big toe was cold it was a sign of approaching childbirth, but the birth would not be imminent until the cold traveled up to the ankle. The extremities become cold, she explained, because much of the blood leaves them at that time and flows to the uterus. The heat collecting in the uterus, resulting from the unusual abundance of the "hot" body fluid, blood, makes the womb uncongenial to the baby, thus aiding in its expulsion.

Since the signs did not point to a quick delivery, and Senani was in no pain or need of moral support, Sapiah decided it would be safe to leave her patient and go to her morning's rubber tapping. We returned twice during the day to check on whether labor had

[153]

begun in earnest, once at 3 P.M. and once at 7 P.M. I noticed that
Senani was wearing bracelet of black twisted wood on her wrist.
She said it was badur wood (*Amorphophallus campanulatus*), given
to her by an Achenese friend to ensure her safety during childbirth. The tubers of badur are poisonous on account of their
needle crystals of oxalate of lime, and its juice is used as a component of dart poison by the Semangs of Perak, one-tenth part
making a poison strong enough to kill a rhinoceros or tiger
(Burkill 1966:140–141). Senani said it was bisa, and so it is. Bisa
can mean both poisonous and powerful, in the sense of a magically effective charm. The badur's empirically poisonous (bisa)
qualities appear to have influenced its symbolically powerful
(bisa) attributes.

At eleven thirty that night a child came to my assistant's house
(next door to mine) to say that Senani was in labor. He awakened
me. I put a sarong and blouse over my nightgown and hopped on
the back of his bicycle. When we arrived, Sapiah was sitting
alongside Senani, gently massaging her abdomen. She had been
there since 11 P.M. She said that it would be some time yet before
the birth. She could tell by feeling Senani's navel: "If it is hard and
raised, birth is imminent." She asked me to touch the navel and
see for myself. It was neither hard nor raised. Sapiah felt the
pulse in Senani's wrist. "If the pulse if fast," she said, "it is a sign
that labor is progressing." Senani's pulse was just a little faster
than normal. Her older brother's wife sat behind her and cradled
Senani's head in her lap. Senani's three-year-old daughter did not
want to sleep and kept coming in and out of the screened-off
room. She did not appear worried or frightened, just very interested in what was taking place. Her aunt told her that she would
soon be the big sister of a new baby. Sapiah asked for the salt
mixture, quietly recited a jampi, and threw it to the four directions and into the space between the floorboards to the ground
below.

The floor on which Senani lay was covered with oilcloth, upon

[154]

which newspapers had been laid. A pail of water stood in a corner of the room, with a cake of soap in a dish alongside, for the midwife to use when washing her hands. Nearby was an empty bucket, used as a receptacle for soiled and dirty cloths. Sapiah had brought along her kit, a covered wicker basket lined with white cloth, in which she kept small bottles filled with habitane-in-spirit for the umbilical stump, dettol (an antiseptic), flavine-in-spirit (in case there are small cuts or tears of the perineum), a pair of scissors, cord to tie the umbilical cord, and absorbent cotton.

Senani lay on her back with her knees flexed, feet close to her buttocks and legs apart. Her sister-in-law placed one hand on each side of Senani's abdomen, above the fundus of the uterus. Senani held her around the hips. She had tied a rolled up sarong above her uterus earlier in the day, to keep the baby from rising.

At 12:55 Sapiah massaged Senani's abdomen, feeling the outline of the uterus. She lifted Senani's sarong to her knees in order to insert a finger into her vagina to ascertain whether the baby's head was already in the vestibule. The three-year-old finally decided to go to sleep on a mat near her mother. Senani began to pray whenever she felt a hard contraction. Between pains she carried on a conversation with the women in the room: Sapiah, her sister-in-law, her mother, and me. The room was lit with two kerosene lamps. The men slept in the outer room on mats that had been spread on the floor. From time to time we women could hear the men snoring and occasionally breaking wind, which always elicited comments and laughter from the women, even from Senani.

For the next two hours Sapiah alternately massaged Senani's abdomen and looked at her vagina. She said that massaging the navel gently encourages the baby to descend. Senani, tiring of her supine position, turned on her side for awhile and then sat up, calling for some coffee. Although she yawned repeatedly, she was alert and in command of the situation.

At 2:45 a little bloody amniotic fluid escaped. Sapiah wiped it away and asked Senani to move so that her head faced southwest, the correct position for the day according to Sapiah's system. Senani complained of pain on the left side of the lower abdomen. Sapiah said it was because the baby was on the right side and would probably be a boy. She asked Senani to grasp her ankles and draw them up close to her buttocks, and encouraged her to bear down with her contractions. Senani's mother entered the room with a basket of baby clothes, and some soft clean old sarongs, which Sapiah tore up for rags. The men, Senani's father, husband, and brother, and my assistant woke up and began to talk in low voices in the outside room. Sapiah placed her finger up Senani's vagina and said that the baby's head was close. Senani's husband, upon hearing his, entered. Sapiah gave him a large piece of bamboo from which he cut a long sharp piece. Sapiah whispered a jampi over it and put it into the clothes basket. She dripped oil into the vaginal opening to make the passage more slippery and massaged Senani's abdomen gently with her oily hands.

By 3:10 Senani had become impatient. She asked Sapiah how much longer and was answered, "Just a little while more." Her father, who had been softly praying in the next room, entered and suggested that they call Pak Su Omar (a respected bomoh), but Sapiah said it would not be necessary. Senani's husband came back and stayed for a few moments, caressing his wife's shoulders. At 3:15 Senani asked her sister-in-law to hold tight over the fundus; at 3:30 there was a gush of amniotic fluid, and at 3:35 the baby's head crowned. Sapiah took it out in a way that reminded me of a head emerging through a turtleneck sweater. She protected the perineum against tearing by pressing a wad of clean cloth against it. She applied upward traction to deliver the posterior shoulder and downward to deliver the anterior shoulder. The baby slipped out easily. It was a boy. Sapiah pointed out to me that her prognosis had been correct.

Sapiah placed the baby on his back, wrapped in a cloth, upon a

folded newspaper. She massaged Senani's abdomen to encourage
expulsion of the afterbirth. As the cord begin to elongate, she
gently pulled on it, wrapping it around her hand. When the
placenta was delivered, she wrapped it in newspaper and turned
her attention once more to the baby. She rubbed his body with
coconut oil to remove the vernix caseosa. A heavy coating of
vernix caseosa, she told me later, is a sure sign that the couple
have been having intercourse during the latter part of pregnancy,
a practice she considers dangerous. She believes the white vernix
caseosa to be an accumulation of semen.

Sapiah rubbed the umbilical cord with heated ashes wrapped in
a little cloth bag. The cord is cold to the touch and must be heated
before it is cut. She put a piece of turmeric under the cord, after
tying it in three places, cut the cord with the piece of sharp
bamboo that had been prepared earlier, and put the end of the
cord still attached to the placenta up to the baby's face for the first
lepas.[16] Then she bathed the baby with soap and warm water in a
basin, using a soft cloth. She rinsed his head with cold water,
because the head is supposed to be naturally hotter than the body.
If it is overheated, sickness or even madness may result. The baby
enjoyed the warm bath but cried when the cold water was poured
on his head. After bathing the baby, Sapiah applied a piece of
absorbent cotton soaked in habitane-in-spirit to the umbilical
stump and covered it with a piece of white cloth, held in place by
an abdominal binder. The bidan dressed the baby in a shirt and
diaper and then wrapped him in a swaddling cloth. Before being
wrapped, the baby's arms and legs must be straightened. The
cloth holds them in place and keeps the baby from exhibiting the
(Moro) startle reaction, which might deplete his semangat.

The midwife handed the clean dressed baby to his grandmother, who touched him lightly with scissors. This was done to
harden his semangat, newly received with the cutting of the
umbilical cord. After the baby had been laid to rest on a small
mattress placed upon a floor mat, covered with a pretty cloth and

surrounded on either side by bolsters, the bidan prepared the afterbirth for burial. She washed it thoroughly in water into which lime juice had been squeezed. After the afterbirth was washed, it was placed inside a half coconut shell, lined with a piece of white cloth. Salt, tamarind, a small piece of absorbent cotton and a bit of white cloth were added. When the midwife had tied the ends of the cloth lining, the "corpse" was ready for burial. Some time within the next few hours the baby's father must bury it beneath a young palm tree, to the accompaniment of prayers for the dead. Salt and tamarind are preservatives and gatekeeping mechanisms, and the bits of cloth and cotton are symbolic representations of the afterbirth's status as semihuman. When Malays bury adult corpses, they use absorbent cotton to close up the orifices and to cover the face. The cotton covers a baby's entire body before it is wrapped in a white winding sheet. The afterbirth is entitled to a decent burial, too, as befits the baby's older sibling. The umbilical cord was not buried with the placenta, but kept for future use. After it has dried it can be ground up and added to water, to make a medicine with which to bathe the baby's eyes, should they become sore. Some people add a bit of dessicated cord to the older siblings' food in the hope that this will decrease family friction; however, the midwife told me that she had done it for her children with no success.

After the placenta had been prepared for burial, the midwife felt Senani's abdomen to see if the uterus was hard. A soft boggy uterus is a danger sign of postpartum hemorrhage, the contingency most feared following delivery. Sapiah massaged the abdomen with coconut oil to expel the "bad" blood of menstruation, accumulated during the many months of pregnancy during which the opening of the womb was glued shut. Senani smiled and held the midwife's ankle affectionately. She changed her sarong and moved to a clean mat and pillow. Her mother handed her a hot tungku stone, which she placed on her abdomen. The midwife cleaned up the debris of childbirth and washed her hands. The father busied himself setting up the "roasting" bed. The grandmother served coffee and steamed cakes. The long night was over. Sapiah, my assistant, and I left for our respective homes, and Senani's family settled down to sleep.

On the way home, my assistant told me that just before the birth took place he awoke to find the hairs on his arms standing on edge, a sign that hantu were about. He thought of telling people to throw rice to chase the spirits away, but decided it was none of his business—yet another example of Malay reluctance to offer advice unless it is specifically requested.

Case no. 2: The birth and death of Asmah's first child

Asmah was a healthy, well-to-do woman in her early twenties. Her family owned a store and a coffee shop. I had visited her often during her pregnancy to collect blood samples and dietary information. Her husband woke me at five o'clock one morning to announce that his wife was in labor. He wanted me to inform the government midwife and drive her to their home. I woke Halimah and waited while she dressed in her white uniform and checked the contents of her delivery kit, an aluminum case. When we arrived, we found that Mak Wah, a bidan kampung, had been there since midnight. Halimah asked Asmah if the baby had moved recently. Asmah was unsure. She felt Asmah's abdomen to see if the head was presenting. She removed her fetal scope from her kit and listened for the baby's heartbeat. She called for hot water to wash her hands, which she scrubbed with her own soap and nail brush and dried on her own hand towel. She gave Asmah an enema, and told her that the baby would descend within an hour, if the birth were to take place that day. Asmah asked Mak Wah to tie a wrapped sarong around her waist to encourage the baby to descend. Mak Wah asked for the salt mixture, recited her jampi and threw it to the four directions and under the floorboards. She rubbed some minyak selusuh, which

[159]

she had prepared at the occasion of Asmah's lenggang perut, on her hands and massaged Asmah's abdomen. Asmah's mother served coffee and cakes. Asmah drank some sweetened coffee but refused the food. Halimah examined Asmah's abdomen again at 7 A.M. and said that the baby would not come until the afternoon, at the earliest. She said she would return later that morning after visiting some nearby patients. Mak Wah, Asmah, and I lay down on mats and pillows to have a nap.

Halimah returned at 9:30. Asmah continued to have mild and irregular contractions. Both midwives sat and talked, occasionally massaging Asmah's abdomen, waiting for labor to begin in earnest. At about 1 P.M. Asmah's mother served lunch. Asmah again would only drink coffee. She felt nauseated. Mak Wah gave her some water with three drops of minyak selusuh to drink. She massaged Asmah's abdomen with some of the treated oil, moistened a cloth with some more, and rubbed it on her vulva. At 2:30, while she was examining Asmah, Halimah noticed meconium escaping from her vagina, a sign of fetal distress. She told Asmah and her husband that this was a bad sign, and recommended that she deliver at the hospital. The husband replied that his wife was perfectly healthy and he saw no reason for her to be moved. Halimah explained that it was the baby she was worried about, not the mother. Neither Asmah nor her husband considered that a valid argument. Halimah told the husband that he would have to sign a statement absolving her of responsibility, since she had recommended hospital delivery but he had not consented. After he signed, Halimah listened for the baby's heartbeat with her fetal scope. She scrubbed her hands again and examined Asmah internally. Her cervix was dilated two fingers. Mak Wah cradled Asmah's head on her lap, placed her hands on Asmah's abdomen, and prayed. Halimah massaged her abdomen, making circular rubbing motions over the navel exactly like those of Sapiah (who claimed to have taught her this technique). Asmah's mother prepared the keras. She and Mak Wah took turns supporting Asmah's head in their laps and pressing above the fundus of her uterus. At 4 P.M. Halimah listened again for the fetal heartbeat. She invited me to listen, too. Although she claimed to hear a beat, I could hear nothing. Asmah's cervix was still dilated only two fingers. At 4:30 Halimah asked me to drive her back to her clinic. She told the family to call her again when the pains were strong.

Asmah's husband came to my house at 9 P.M. that night and asked me to pick up Halimah. When we arrived, we found that Pak Cu, a bomoh who specializes in difficult labors, had been called. Pak Cu treats no other conditions. He uses Arabic sentences from the Koran in place of the usual Malay jampi. Asmah's head rested on his lap. She put her arms around his back with every contraction. Asmah's religion teacher, with whom she had studied Koran as a child in Kelantan, had sent her a bottle of air tawar to use during labor. She took sips from time to time during the next few hours and used it on a cloth to refresh her face. Halimah opened her delivery kit and spread the contents on a clean white towel. Her kit contained the following:

1 kidney basin and 2 smaller bowls
2 clamps for umbilical cord
1 cord scissors
1 syringe and 2 needles
enema set
mucus extractor
fetal scope
baby's spring balance scale
thermometer
urethral catheter
forceps for lifting bowls
sterilizer container
sterile cotton swabs, gauze
soap, nailbrush, and towel
plastic apron
plastic square
2 ampules of ergometrine

[161]

1 bottle of Panadol (analgesic)
1 bottle of Dettol (antiseptic)
1 bottle of flavine-in-spirit
1 bottle of habitane-in-spirit
1 bottle of cord ligatures
1 bottle of eyedrops

Halimah scrubbed her hands and cleaned Asmah's perineal area with dettol. She asked Asmah's mother to bring clothes in which to wrap the baby. Night was falling and little kerosene lamps were lit. Mak Wah took Pak Cu's place at Asmah's head. She moistened Asmah's long hair with the minyak selusuh and wiped her abdomen with the oiled hair. She took some lime from a box containing the ingredients for betel chewing and rubbed it on Asmah's abdomen. Halimah sat at one side of Asmah's flexed legs and I sat at the other. She dripped coconut oil into Asmah's vagina just as Sapiah had done. Mak Wah advised Asmah to move so that her head faced west.

Asmah was in pain, but she did not cry or scream. She said, "It's been going on for such a long time," and asked how much longer it would be. The women advised her to pray. She asked for Pak Cu, who had been sitting in the outside room. He massaged her abdomen with minyak selusuh and recited passages from the Koran. At 10:30 Asmah began to push every two minutes. She asked for her husband, who came into the room to sit by her side and hold her hand. Her mother served coffee again, but this time Asmah did not drink. By eleven, Asmah's contractions had once more become irregular. At 11:25 a second bomoh arrived. He recited a jampi and threw rice to repel any noxious spiritual presences. By now everyone was yawning. The children (Asmah's siblings and cousins) had already fallen asleep in the outside room. One woke up and cried and was quickly comforted by one of the women.

Mak Wah told Asmah's husband to step over his wife's body three times. Perhaps labor has been prolonged because of her

behavior during pregnancy. Halimah did another internal examination and said that delivery would soon take place. The second
bomoh came back into the room, said another jampi and threw
some more rice. He gave Asmah a cloth which had been treated
with benzoin fumes and incantations to tie around her left hand.

At 12:30 A.M. Halimah fell asleep. About 1 A.M., Mak Wah
woke her up. She did a vaginal examination and asked Mak Wah
to wake her again when she saw the baby's head crown. By 2 A.M.
the baby's black hair could be seen at the end of the birth passage,
but then it withdrew from sight. Mak Wah woke Halimah and
told Asmah's parents to open all the doors and windows. The
second bomoh came in and recited another jampi. Halimah told
Asmah to sit up and try to urinate. Mak Wah said it would be wise
to move her into another room. She was beginning to feel the
presence of hantu. I asked whether they would like me to call for
an ambulance. Asmah's husband and mother wanted to wait a
while longer. Halimah said that she thought an ambulance
should be called if the baby was not delivered soon. It started to
rain, a steady torrential downpour heralding the arrival of the
monsoon season. Asmah was moved into another room near the
kitchen. At 2:45 the family agreed that it was time to call for an
ambulance. I went out to turn my car around, but when I re-
entered the house, Halimah said, "Wait, the baby is ready to come
out." For the last hour the top of its head could be seen, approaching the opening of the vagina and retreating. At 2:55 the
baby was born. As its head emerged, we could see that the umbilical cord was looped three times around its neck. Halimah quickly
unlooped the cord, clamped and cut it.

She lifted the baby out. It was painfully thin and dehydrated, its
ribs were showing, its stomach was sunken, and its body was limp.
Mak Wah spat several times in the baby's direction.[17] Halimah
massaged the baby's back, but it did not respond. The afterbirth
was delivered. The umbilical cord was green, the placenta green
and black, the amniotic fluid had turned black. Asmah's mother

said "*Tak apa-apa.*" (It's nothing, it's all right). The phrase was repeated by almost everyone. Asmah echoed, "*Tak apa-apa.*" No one cried. The only silent ones were myself and Halimah. Mak Wah said that she could feel the hantu pushing the baby back into Asmah's body for an hour before it finally emerged. She said that the hantu had been able to suck the baby's blood because its body had been weakened by the looped cord.

Asmah was very tired. She lay back and closed her eyes. Halimah washed the dead baby, wrapped it in cloth and laid it down on the small mattress which had been prepared to receive a live child. I placed mosquito netting over it. It was to remain there until the family had rested from its ordeal. The following day it was buried in the cemetery.

Halimah washed the afterbirth and prepared it for burial. Mak Wah prepared bath water with "hot" leaves for Asmah while her husband and stepfather got the "roasting bed" ready. Asmah's mother served more drinks. It was 5 A.M., exactly twenty-four hours since we had first arrived. Halimah asked me to drive her home. Mak Wah stayed on to clean up the debris.

Certain norms guided the behavior of the actors in the two cases I have recounted: the wishes of the mother were a primary consideration, her feminine modesty was respected, and her emotions were not given free rein in the face of pain and even death. The bidan's ritual activities during the birth of Senani's child were the bare minimum necessary for a normal birth: she threw the salt mixture, prepared the afterbirth for burial, and performed a preliminary lepas for the baby. Ritual activities increase considerably when labor is protracted or when there are unusual circumstances connected with the birth, as in Asmah's case. In addition to the normal precautions, the bidan rubbed minyak selusuh on Asmah's stomach, hair, and vulva and gave her some to drink. She bathed her face with air tawar, which Asmah also drank. She rubbed lime on her abdomen to make her womb "hotter" and therefore less attractive to the baby, following humoral rather than magical theory. She advised Asmah's husband to step over his wife's body to reverse the negative effects of her behavior during pregnancy. Two bomoh were also called in on the case, one who specialized in childbirth and employed only Koranic sentences, and a second who uses Malay jampi and who prepared an amulet for the laboring woman. When none of these treatments had the desired effect, the midwife suggested that Asmah move to another room to escape the hantu's influence, and requested that all doors and windows be opened.

Invoking the laws of sympathetic magic by opening doors and cupboards, loosening the mother's hair, and leaving windows wide open (described as normal procedure in rural Malay births by Wylde 1957:131; Winstedt 1951:106; Chen 1975:105) is not a usual feature of childbirth in Merchang. When a sick woman is treated by a bomoh, her hair must hang down to allow the sickness to escape from her body, but while she is in the throes of labor her hair is swept up to keep her cool and comfortable. Neither cupboards nor doors are deliberately opened for normal births. Since few houses have internal doors, the room in which birth is to occur is partitioned off from the rest of the house by means of a cloth hung over a string. Windows in the delivery room are usually left closed to protect the mother's modesty, and mats or cloths are placed against walls that have spaces or chinks that might afford passersby a glimpse of the drama within. On stifling hot days, windows may be opened a crack, but the women make sure that the shutters or cloths are arranged so as to preserve decorum. Except in unusual and dangerous circumstances, considerations of feminine modesty outweigh the possible benefits that a magical correspondence between open windows and open wombs might confer. Asmah's ordeal was the only occasion on which I witnessed doors and windows opened to facilitate birth.

Malay women are encouraged to pray during labor and are strongly discouraged from crying or screaming. On one occasion a young woman giving birth to her first child was lightly slapped on the face when she cried out. The assembled women asked her if she had no shame, to act in that manner. In many respects this is a useful *adat* (custom in the widest sense of the word). Concentration on prayer rather than pain may lead a woman away from anxieties that can interfere with her uterine functions. If incipient hysteria is cut off in its beginnings, and a satisfactory alternative substituted, it may be beneficial for the outcome of labor. The prohibition against exhibiting strong emotions is a salient feature of rural Malay life.

During the course of a survey, I asked people whether they thought that strong emotions could affect physical health. I was almost invariably told, "I never have any strong emotions." At the funeral of Rohani's baby, I was the only person crying. My assistant told me that when his wife almost died bringing forth his firstborn, a stillbirth, he did not shed a single tear. The reaction to the tragic outcome of Asmah's protracted labor was, "It's all right, it's nothing." This denial of emotions takes its toll. Most of the conditions treated by Malay shamans are classified by them as sakit berangin, a disease whose etiology is the frustration of talent, character, and desires.

THE MIDWIFE AS MEDICAL PRACTITIONER

Although, in the cases presented above, the normal birth was attended only by a traditional midwife while the stillbirth was attended by both government midwife and bidan kampung, I in no way mean to suggest that the government midwife can be held responsible for the tragic outcome. She recognized the signs of fetal distress and recommended hospital delivery to the parents, but she was in no position to compel them to follow her recommendation. Her behavior was not only congruent with rural Malay standards of courtesy and noninterference but was also strategically correct, given her position within the community.

Giving Birth in a Malay Village

Had she insisted or tried to bully the family into following her suggestion, she would have encountered opposition which might easily have spread and generalized to other potential patients and their families. As I pointed out earlier, villagers do not consider the government midwife's services absolutely essential. A domineering government midwife might soon find herself persona non grata.

Ignoring the bidan's ritual function and considering her only in her role of medical practitioner, we find there are many points of similarity between the performance of the government midwife and that of the bidan kampung. Both provide moral support and encouragement to their patients, both deliver the baby in the same manner, both massage the woman's abdomen before delivery to soothe her and after the baby is born to facilitate expulsion of the placenta. Both know the signs of placental separation and are careful to note the elongation of the umbilical cord before they slowly and carefully pull it to assist in the delivery of the afterbirth. Both clean, bathe, and dress the baby.

Their differences seem primarily a matter of emphasis rather than true divergence. The point of difference stressed by the villagers credits the bidan kampung with always being available and staying with her patient from the onset of labor through its conclusion. They frequently criticized the government midwife for being unavailable during the night and while her clinic was in progress. They also complained that she would not stay with her patient for more than an hour or two, and accused her of trying to speed up her patient's delivery by putting her fingers up into the birth canal.

The last complaint has no basis whatever in reality. It is clear from my accounts of births attended by government and traditional midwives that both do several vaginal examinations during the course of labor. Halimah, being trained to gauge cervical dilatation, examines farther up the vestibule than Sapiah, who merely wants to ascertain whether the baby has begun its descent

[167]

down the birth canal. Although the availability of the government midwife was a real problem, because she was afraid of going out alone at night, the villager's estimation of the bidan kampung's availability was somewhat illusory. As we have seen in chapter 5, village midwives do not make a conscious effort to be within constant reach of their clients, but go about their daily activities. The difference between the relative unavailability of the government and traditional midwives is due primarily to the fact that there is only one of the former and many of the latter. If any particular bidan kampung is unavailable, another can be called. The government midwife, as the sole representative of her calling in the parish, is highly visible and her role cannot easily be carried out by a substitute.

Complaints about the government midwife's not seeing her patients through their entire labors and deliveries have two dimensions. The first is her time allocation. She must attend to many duties besides the one at hand. If, in her judgment, the patient will not deliver within the next couple of hours, she may decide that it is safe to leave her temporarily. This, as we have seen, was also true of Sapiah, yet no one complained about her. The reason for this difference in patients' attitudes is the second dimension of this problem. Sapiah, with her many years of experience, had extremely good judgment about the imminence of birth. In all the time I spent in Merchang, I never observed or heard of a case where she left her patient only to find upon her return that she had given birth unattended. This was not uncommon, however, in Halimah's case. On four occasions where I was present and several others that were reported to me, Halimah left her patient, assuring her that she would not deliver until much later, and the woman delivered within the following hour. This was not owing to any laziness or unconcern on Halimah's part, as villagers supposed. Where circumstances were clearly abnormal, as in the case of Asmah, Halimah spent as much as eight consecutive hours in attendance. The difference, then, was not so much in the length of time spent at the patient's side as it was in the judgment of when it was safe to leave her unattended.

The point of difference stressed by the medical establishment in Trengganu was the government midwife's sterile procedures and the traditional midwife's lack of them. As noted in the accounts above, both Sapiah and Halimah washed their hands before and after vaginal examinations. Halimah used hot boiled water and scrubbed with a nail brush, while Sapiah only used well water and soap. Both used cloths to protect the perineum against tearing, but Halimah used a sterile pad while Sapiah used clean old pieces of sarong. Halimah's instruments were sterilized, while Sapiah usually used a clean but unsterilized pair of scissors to cut the umbilical cord. Halimah used a bulb syringe to remove mucus from a baby's airways, while Sapiah used her own mouth. Halimah's sterile procedures broke down, however, during the last part of labor. Probably following Sapiah's example, she dripped ordinary coconut oil into her patient's vagina.

Both villagers and bidan kampung found Halimah's delivery kit impressive and enviable. She regularly gave her patient an enema if there was enough time before the delivery, thus obviating the frequent unaesthetic mess which the bidan kampung were accustomed to cleaning up during labor. However, the standard enema customarily given to women in labor by hospital-trained medical attendants has been shown to cause electrolyte imbalances (Birnbaum 1978:108). The bidan kampung admired the way Halimah clamped and cut the umbilical cord before the placenta was delivered, and they would have liked to have been able to copy her actions. Delay in cutting the cord, however, has been demonstrated to add an appreciable amount of iron to the baby's store by favoring maximal drainage of blood from the placenta into the baby's body (McLean 1951:136). Moreover, early clamping of the umbilical cord has been shown to lengthen the third stage of labor, and increase the likelihood of maternal hemorrhage, retained placenta, or the retention of placental fragments (Botha 1968:30−33).

On balance it appears that some of the newer procedures are

conducive to the greater health and safety of the baby, that is, sterile scissors used to cut the cord, avoiding the threat of neonatal tetanus, while others introduce the possibility of iatrogenesis, for instance, cutting the cord before the end of the third stage of labor.

Halimah's strength lay in her recognition of danger signals during labor and her ability to summon help via the ambulance. Her professional strength, however, was turned to impotence in the face of her patients' refusal to heed her advice.

The most serious accusation made against bidan kampung by medical authorities is that they contribute to maternal death by attempting to expel the fetus forcibly if labor is prolonged (Chen 1974–1975:341; Siti Hasmah 1968:6; Sambhi 1968:347; Thambu 1971:294). This procedure will not rupture the uterus if the cervix has fully dilated. If prolongation of labor is, however, owing to obstruction, such as abnormal presentation of the baby, or disproportion, pressing down very strongly on the uterus can cause it to rupture, resulting in death for the mother and child unless emergency laparotomy is carried out. The pressure must be that of "extreme violence" (Thambu 1971:294) "so brutal as to cause bruising of the gut" (Sambhi 1968:348). Such strength is not usual in a Malay woman, so "a few strong men have [to be] called in by the Bomoh midwife to apply pressure on the abdomen and uterus with the view of pushing the baby out" (Sambhi 1968:347). Although Dr. Siti Hasmah says that obstructed labor, combined with pressure on the uterus exerted by bidan kampung "is frequently the cause of maternal death" (1968:6), the figures from the General Hospital at Kuantan, covering all cases admitted to the Department of Obstetrics and Gynecology for the period January 1968 to December 1969, show four cases per year (Thambu 1971:293). On the basis of this data, Thambu concludes that "rupture of the uterus is a rare condition" (1971:294).

None of the traditional midwives I observed pressed down violently on the parturient woman's uterus or called in strong men to do so for her, although I was present at several protracted labors. They did massage the abdomen, particularly the navel area, both in an effort to ease the woman's discomfort and in the belief that it would speed up delivery, but the massage was done gently and carefully. A woman in labor customarily lies with her head in the lap of a female relative, who presses on her diaphragm while she grasps her kin around the waist from behind, but the pressure exerted is not enough to cause damage. If the woman in labor objects to this procedure, it is not performed or is discontinued. No doubt such violent treatment and dire results can be attributed to some bidan kampung. There are levels of intelligence and competence in any field, and the lengthy training of a bidan is no more a guarantee of excellence in all midwives than a medical degree is an assurance that a particular physician possesses the competence that such a degree implies. Every group of medical practitioners provides its patients with both valuable care and a certain measure of iatrogenic harm. To characterize the entire group by the standards of its worst practitioners, however, would be grossly unfair.

A theme running through rural Malay beliefs and practices connected with childbirth is that of flexibility and accommodation. According to a popular saying, "If you are giving birth, you should listen to the midwife" (*Kalau kita beranak, ikut kata bidan*), but she is listened to because of her authority, accumulated over years of successful practice, and not because of any power to compel behavior. The mother's comfort and wishes must be respected. The bidan only assists; the mother has the final decision. If she wants to lie on her side or sit up, and the birth is not imminent, there is nothing to prevent her from doing so. If she wants to eat or drink during labor, she may. If she doesn't want to wear a sash during labor, she may discard it. If she objects to pressure being exerted on her abdomen, it will be stopped. The only rules she must follow are not to stand during the last phase of labor so as to avoid the possibility of the baby's emerging rapidly and dropping on its head, and to keep her legs spread during delivery, for obvious reasons.

Even in the case of protracted or abnormal labor, the role of the parturient woman is not usurped. Although one or more bomoh may be called in, they do not become hero shamans or physicians, but remain merely her assistants and attendants. Bomoh and bidan may be thanked for their efforts, and their assistance is highly valued, but parents, and not they, are congratulated on the birth of a child.

Malay treatment of abnormal labors, and the theory behind it, have both positive and negative aspects. The bidan's reassurances and use of magical paraphernalia, and the bomoh's incantations, may change the laboring woman's biochemical and physiological responses, aiding her in the successful completion of her task. However, lack of recognition of fetal distress on the part of bidan kampung, and Asmah's refusal to avail herself of the benefits of hospital delivery, illustrate a defect in Malay traditional childbirth practices. Had Asmah and her family understood the significance of escaping meconium and the necessity for immediate medical intervention, the baby's life might have been saved.

Every society has priorities that shape the ideology and conduct of childbirth. In America, mindful of possible dangers to the mother and child, we treat birth as a potentially life-threatening illness. For the mother's safety, she must be placed in the hands of an expert whose decisions, although they may be open to discussion along the way, are ultimately final. While this may minimize certain risks, it undoubtedly diminishes the mother's autonomy. Rural Malays view childbirth as a normal event in every woman's life which, however, may infrequently imperil her well-being. The dangers of childbirth are not allowed to erode her autonomy—her decisions are respected, even when they may lead to her death. On one occasion, a mother was told by the government midwife that she might die unless she delivered at the hospital.

Since she was living alone, her husband having gone to work outside the kampung and no other relative within easy reach, she said she preferred to die at home rather than go to the hospital by herself. None of her neighbors attempted to change her mind. When my assistant noticed my concern, he said it was nobody's business but her own: if she wanted to die, then let her die. Fortunately, she did not die, but if she had, the responsibility would have been entirely hers.

Whether one takes the view that traditional Malay childbirth practices foolishly expose the mother and child to unnecessary risks, or sees them as procedures that allow a woman to take command during the most important hours of her life, the essential difference between childbirth in America and childbirth in Merchang is clear: American women are delivered by obstetricians; Malay women give birth.

· 7 ·

The Postpartum Period

The postpartum period is the liminal stage in a woman's passage through the rite of childbirth. As in all such transitional stages, the person on the threshold is in an extremely vulnerable position and must be segregated from her community. For the new mother in Merchang, the segregation is behavioral rather than physical.

Her spirit as well as her body is in danger, and the two are closely entwined, since a weakened body is a poor fortress for the spirit within, and a depleted spirit weakens the body still further. The bidan must be adept at dealing with both eventualities, but she will not hesitate to call for reinforcements if a problem goes beyond her capabilities. A bomoh may be brought in when a problem is diagnosed as stemming from intrusion by the spirit world. If the problem involves serious postpartum hemorrhage or infection, the government midwife may be consulted and the services of the hospital utilized.

With the expulsion of the baby and the subsequent loss of blood, the "hot" body fluid, the new mother enters into a "cold" state that lasts until her ceremonial release, approximately forty days after the birth of her child. This humoral belief is supported by physiological evidence, as illustrated by the following advice given to nursing students in an American manual on pregnancy (Anderson et al. 1974–1975:I, 246):

> During this first critical hour of the fourth stage of labor [immediately after delivery], the mother may experience a shaking chill. This reaction does not commonly result in an elevation of body temperature nor is it associated with any type of infection. The mother should be covered with a blanket and, if alert, can at this time be given warm tea to drink.

If the woman has hyperventilated for an extended period the chill reaction can be quite severe. My second child was induced by the administration of pitocin, a drug that causes stronger uterine contractions than normal, faster paced but with shorter relaxation periods between contractions (Montagu 1977:594). This change in the normal rhythm of contractions, coupled with a desire to avoid all analgesia or anesthesia, made it necessary for me to inhale and exhale great gusts of air, one following close upon the other. After the baby was born, I became ice cold and the tips of my fingers and toes were bright blue. It was necessary to cover me with piles of blankets and monitor my blood pressure for over an hour after the birth.

The cold produced by an abnormal labor can be quite dramatic, but even the transitory chill described in the nurses' manual would be enough to convince a rural Malay that the new mother's body must be warmed both inside and out to bring it back to its normal state. Immediately following delivery, the bidan kampung bathes her in water that has been warmed on the stove and heated still further by the addition of "hot" and fragrant leaves. These leaves are humorally rather than thermally hot. Some of the more popular are *daun kemudu* (*Morinda citrifolia*), *daun kuau* (*Peristrophe acuminata*), and *pandan wangi* (*Pandanus odurus*), but any hot leaves will suffice. Malays ordinarily bathe in cool well water, even during the chilly monsoon season. For a cold new mother and her infant, however, the bath water must be heated.

[175]

Skeat (1972:334–335) considered bathing the new mother to be a rite of purification. The postparturient Malay mother, however, cannot be purified by a bath. According to Muslim doctrine, she will remain in a state of ritual impurity until the lochia have ceased to flow. Since postpartal vaginal discharge will cease after three to six weeks, the new mother will probably become ritually pure in Islam while she is still in the transitional stage of the rite of passage.

After she has been bathed, the new mother's abdomen is rubbed with a paste made of ginger, garlic, tamarind, and lime (*kapur*) (some people use only a mixture of salt and turmeric). These "hot" substances are supposed to help shrink the uterus. A long sash is then wound tightly around her waist to help her regain her shape.

While she is being bathed, the men of her family set up the *salaian*, known in the literature as the "roasting bed," and the women prepare the tungku, a smooth flat stone heated on the hearth and wrapped in cloth, about the size of a hot water bag and used for a similar purpose. The mother places it on her abdomen to add heat and to relieve discomfort. Some bidan kampung advise their patients not to use the tungku right away, as it might dry up the "bad" blood, preventing it from being expelled.

When the men have set up the salaian, a simple wooden frame with boards across its width on which an old floor mat is placed, the new mother leaves the floor to lie upon her "roasting bed." Beneath the salaian or, less often, alongside it, a large pot or box containing a small wood fire is placed. The heat of the fire is thought to dry up the lochia faster (reducing the days of ritual impurity), to cause the blood to circulate faster (since the mother's cold state slows down the circulation of the blood), to encourage the rapid involution of the uterus, close up the cervix (discouraging the possibility of pregnancy in the near future), and aid the mother in regaining her youthful figure and tight vagina. This last item is of considerable importance to a Malay wife, many of

[176]

whom have remarked to me that when the vagina becomes loose, so does the husband's attachment to his wife.

Postparturient Malay women do not neglect their internal coldness. Most of them begin to take heating medicines soon after delivery. However, just as many bidan kampung feel that premature use of the tungku can dry up the "dirty" blood and cause the uterus to swell, so, too, they fear that the ingestion of medicine that is too hot immediately after delivery may cause similar problems. Most women avoid this danger by taking a mixture of two roots, *sepang* (*Caesalpinia sappan*) and *kederang* (*Caesalpinia* sp.) for a period of from three to twenty days after delivery. These roots, which are considered to be "pleasantly warm," are boiled in a quantity of water. At least three glasses of the liquid are drunk each day. The period during which very hot root medicines are avoided is not dictated by any set rule but varies with the individual mother. When she feels ready, she switches from sepang kederang to *akar kayu* (the generic name for root medicines, but in this case referring to the hot postpartum mixtures). Although sepang kederang are easy to find and are usually collected by a member of the family, many people purchase their supply of akar kayu from a bidan, bomoh, or other person skilled at finding the ingredients. Sometimes called "medicine of a hundred ingredients" (*ubat seratus bangsa*), the actual number is closer to ten. Sapiah's supply of akar kayu for postpartum cases contained the following:

susu harimau (*Polystictus rhinocerotis*)
tongkat Ali (*Euricoma longifolia*)
kacip Fatimah (*Labisia pothoina*)
misai Ali (unidentified)
kubur melawan (*Plumeria?*)
akar teja (*Cinnamomun* sp.)
repoh gunung (literally mountain shrub, unidentified)
janggut Ali (*Panicum sarmentosum*)
garok (*Willughbeia coriacea*)
sireh hutan (*Piper caninum*)

[177]

Besides having the humoral quality of "heat," many of these ingredients have names that are symbolically evocative. *Susu harimau* means tiger's milk, and what could be better for restoring a person's strength? *Kubur melawan* means the grave's adversary. *Tongkat Ali*, *misai Ali*, and *janggut Ali* (Ali's staff, moustache, and beard)—all make reference to Muhammad's son-in-law, while *kacip Fatimah* (Fatimah's areca nut slicer) refers to Ali's wife, the daughter of the Prophet. Together they are regarded by Malays as the perfect husband and ideal wife.

Although most women take akar kayu, some substitute or add a complex electuary manufactured under the name of Ma'jun, which is sold by bidan kampung, who buy it wholesale from itinerant peddlers.

Penicillin, which can be purchased in tablet form without a prescription at local stores, is occasionally used for its extremely hot qualities. One new mother took a single penicillin tablet because the pains in her abdomen were diagnosed by the bidan as being caused by blood clots formed during the birth process, when air entered the temporarily open womb. The extreme heat of the penicillin, she thought, could liquify the clotted blood. Taking too many tablets, however, is believed to dry up the blood and cause the abdomen to swell.

Besides her own internal and external application of heat, the new mother's body heat is increased by the bidan kampung in her role as masseuse. She massages her patient from the top of her head to the tips of her toes for about an hour on each of three successive mornings following delivery, to improve her circulation and muscle tone and heal the internal wounds caused by childbirth. The bidan pays special attention to the mother's breasts, massaging them carefully to encourage the milk supply. All massage is done by hand, and not with a tungku stone, as has been reported by Wylde (1957:132).

Even those women who have dispensed with the services of a bidan kampung during delivery, or who have delivered at the

[178]

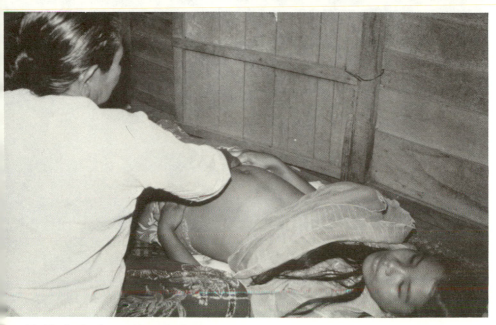

A **midwife** checks the position of a fetus.

A cylinder of palas leaves is rolled across a prospective mother's abdomen.

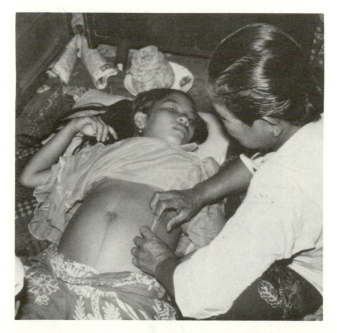

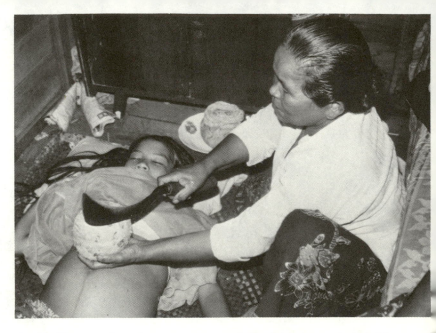

A midwife pretends to cleave a coconut, symbolic of the pregnant womb. The second coconut, partially covered by cord, is the *keras*.

A mother-to-be passes through the cord that forms part of the *keras*, symbolic of birth and rebirth.

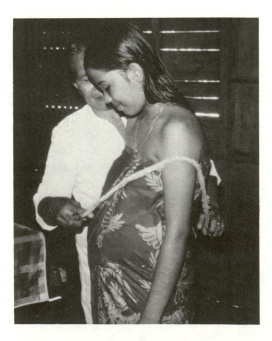

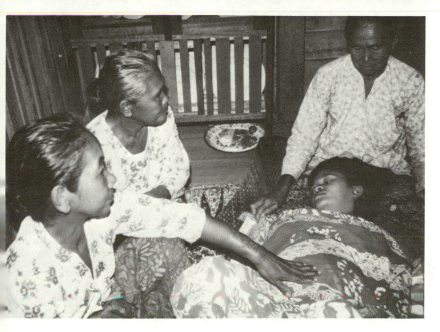

A **woman** in labor rests on her mother's lap, while a midwife massages her abdomen.

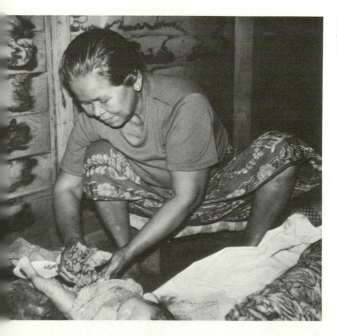

A **midwife** heats an umbilical cord with a bag of warmed sand before cutting it.

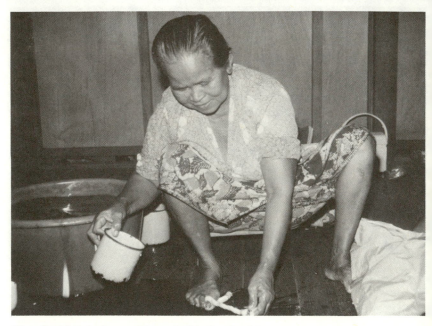

The afterbirth is thoroughly washed before burial.

The afterbirth is placed in a coconut shell "coffin," lined with a "winding sheet."

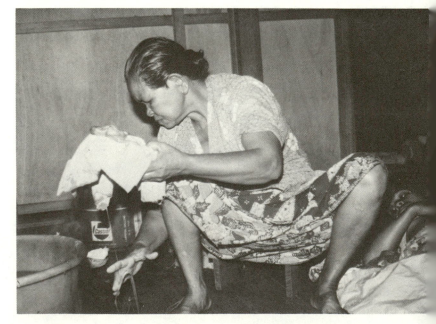

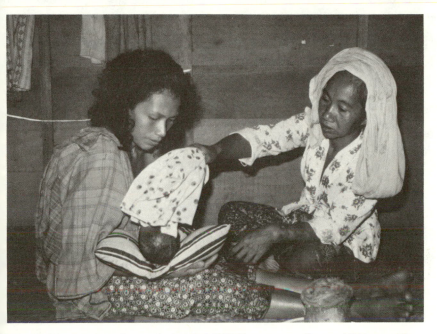

midwife recites incantations and wipes baleful influences away from a child born with
umbilical cord around its neck.

hile a new mother is massaged, the midwife's young daughter looks on to learn.

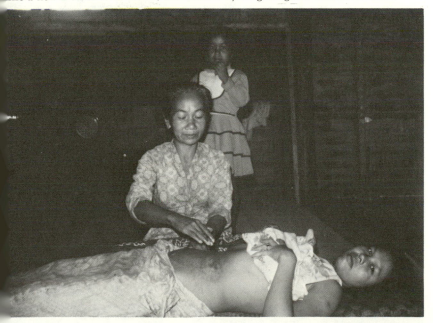

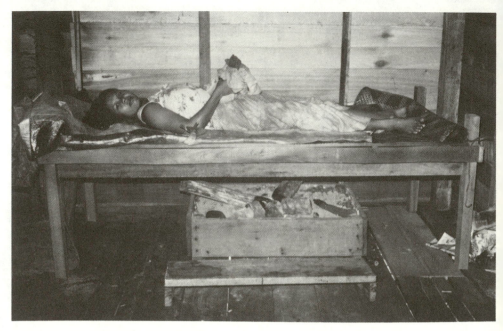

A new mother rests on the "roasting bed" and warms her abdomen with a *tungku* stone.

A chicken is encouraged to scratch among the ashes under the "roasting bed" to absorb evil influences.

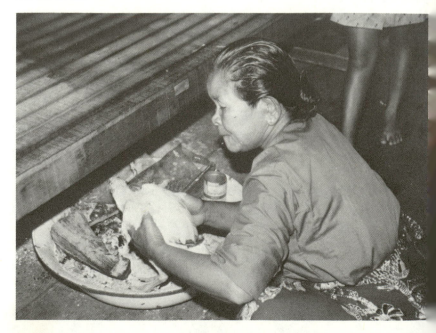

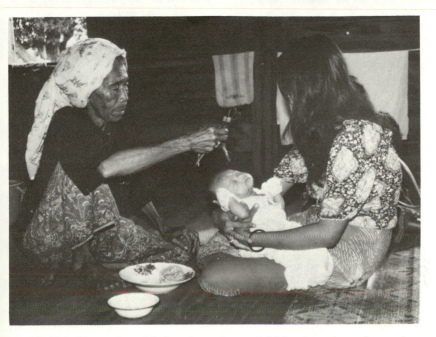

A midwife holds a "releaser" before the mother and child as she recites an incantation.

The postpartum ritual over, a midwife relaxes. The white spot on her forehead is *tepung tawar*.

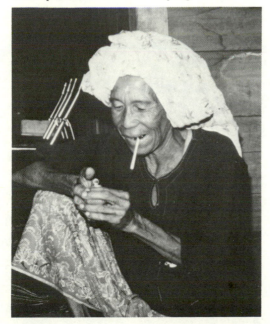

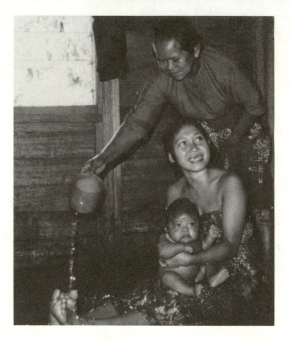

A **mother** and child receive a
purifying bath. Note the *tepung
tawar* on the baby's forehead.

A baby girl is prepared for clitorodotomy (cutting off a tiny portion
of the clitoral hood).

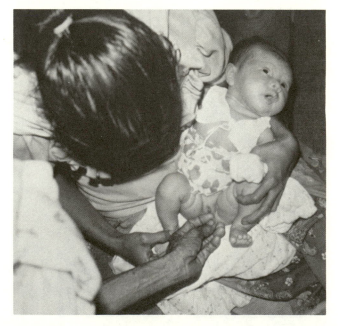

hospital, will not forego this relaxing postpartum massage. Higher education does not appear to diminish faith in the necessity for and efficacy of Malay postpartum traditions, on the east coast. One of my friends in Kelantan, who had received her Master's degree in biology from Columbia University, was married to a well-known doctor and taught science in a prestigious school. She delivered her first child at the state hospital. When she returned to her kampung, however, she came under the care of a traditional midwife, observed the postpartum food restrictions and used the "roasting bed."

Variations in the amount of time new mothers in Merchang spent on the salaian or used the tungku varied widely between those who never did either to those who stayed on the salaian day and night (see tables 10 and 11). About the same number of women stayed on the *salaian* for only an hour or two during the day as those who did so all day long. During the night, the fire was banked and most women slept above the embers. Besides this individual variation, there were also seasonal variations. Women welcomed the opportunity of lying over a small fire during the chilly monsoon season, whereas in the hot dry season they were more likely to limit their observance of this custom. Women who have just delivered their first babies spend more time on the salaian than those with larger families. This is not because the primapara is considered any "colder" than other mothers, but because the demands made on her time by her older children prevent the multipara from lying on the "roasting bed" as long as she might like.

The use of the salaian has been criticized by a number of outside observers from the early days of this century to very recent times. According to Skeat (1972:342), because of the "extreme heat" of the salaian, "on one occasion a poor woman was brought to the point of death . . . and would have died if she had not been rescued by the kind interposition of the Civil Assistant-Surgeon; the excessive excitement caused by the heat was so

[179]

TABLE 10
USE OF THE SALAIAN DURING DAYLIGHT HOURS

	Percent	*Number*
Never	2	(2)
Night only	7	(6)
One hour a day	14	(12)
Two hours	14	(12)
Three hours	14	(12)
Four hours	3.5	(3)
Five hours	6	(5)
Six hours	3.5	(3)
Seven hours	3.5	(3)
Eight hours	1	(1)
Nine hours	1	(1)
Ten hours	3.5	(3)
All day	26	(22)

N = 85

TABLE 11
USE OF THE TUNGKU STONE

	Percent	*Number*
Never	5	(4)
One hour a day	14	(12)
Two hours	25	(21)
Three hours	29	(25)
Four hours	7	(6)
Five hours	2	(2)
Six hours	6	(5)
Seven hours	1	(1)
Eight hours	2	(2)
Nine hours	1	(1)
All day	7	(6)

N = 85

over-powering that aberration of mind ensued which continued for several months." More modern commentators do not implicate the salaian as a cause of madness, but a factor in acute congestive cardiac failure (Chen 1974−1975:344) and failure of lactation (Whyte 1974:64). Since, as Chen points out (1973:204), there have not been any studies to show that there is a significant degree of poor lactation in those who "roast" compared with those who do not, and the only ground for implicating the Malay salaian in congestive cardiac failure is its similarity to a form of puerperal roasting in Northern Nigeria (Chen 1974−1975:345), one wonders why this practice is condemned, while many forms of heat treatment in other cultures (e.g., sauna, Turkish bath, American Indian sweat lodge, diathermy) have been accepted as having validity.

One possibility is that the word has gained in force during its translation into English. *Salai* is a word used "generally of processes where prolonged exposure to heat (not extreme heat) are required" (Wilkinson 1959:1005). Translating salaian as "roasting" ups the temperature considerably in the minds of English speakers. It might, with more accuracy, be called *warming* or *heating* the mother. Another possible reason for the condemnation of the salaian is the reaction of the English to the heat of the tropics. English families, who considered the musim kemarau unbearably hot, retired to the cool hill stations during the summer months. Some English families lived in the hills all year round to escape the heat, the wives and children staying up on the hill while the husbands descended daily by cable car to their work below. To an Englishman, even one who played soccer in the noonday sun, the idea of deliberately adding heat in the infernally hot tropics must have seemed the height of madness and superstition. Modern Malaysian scientists appear to have inherited some of the prejudices of their English intellectual forebears, although they may not recognize their roots.

One sees again and again in the literature references to high

[181]

heats and constantly replenished fires, above which the new mother is supposed to spend most of her waking and all of her sleeping hours. Had I never seen a salaian, I would have been under the impression that it featured a roaring fire, and that the new mother was constrained to suffer its discomfort in all seasons—a virtual prisoner of custom. In actuality, the fires of the salaian in Merchang were quite low during the day and banked at night. Most women said that the heat was soothing and comfortable except in the musim kemarau, when time on the salaian was cut to a minimum. Rather than being slaves to custom, many women were manipulators. For example, although the usual length of the puerperium is forty days, some women, bored with the salaian and eager to be released from postpartum restrictions, elected to have the ceremony of release performed after thirty-five or thirty-six days.

The tungku, too, has not escaped criticism. Siti Hasmah (1968:9) wrote that "usually" the tungku is "so over-heated that the skin of the abdomen is burnt literally black and the muscles underneath lose their resilience and ability to contract. The abdominal wall becomes loose, thin and dry and quite incapable of assisting in expelling the foetus at future births." Although this may be the case in other parts of Malaysia, it was not so in Merchang. Since only 5 percent of the women I surveyed never used the tungku, one might expect that the other 95 percent would show evidence of abdominal burns and be unable to give birth without surgical intervention to any children after the first. However, of the many women I observed during childbirth and massaged thereafter, a number of them grand multiparas, none showed any sign of abdominal burns. Despite the widespread use of the tungku, the average number of children in a Merchang family is five, but thirteen is not unheard of. Cesarian, or any other hospital delivery, is a great rarity. In Merchang, the use of the tungku has not interfered with normal vaginal deliveries. I have touched tungku stones wrapped in cloth as they were given to new mothers and found them equal in heat to a rubber hot water bag, which must also be wrapped in cloth to be bearable if filled with very hot water.

Even the rest from hard work which is a feature of the Malay postpartum period (and found in most known societies) has been criticized. Wylde (1957:132) says that, due to the lack of exercise, "the mother's muscles lose tone with the result that at each subsequent pregnancy her physical condition deteriorates." Those who have witnessed the energy and seen the trim figures of Malay mothers of nine and ten children will find it hard to give this statement credence.

What emerges from this discussion is that outside observers, speaking in the name of science, have condemned Malay traditional childbirth practices on the flimsiest of evidence. This theme will be repeated and enlarged in the discussion of postpartum food restrictions.

POSTPARTUM FOOD RESTRICTIONS

Early folklorists were careful to take note of Malay postpartum food restrictions as part of the study of the popular religion of the people, and more recent investigators have been concerned with these pantang as a contributory factor in ill health. Skeat (1972: 343–344) mentions as forbidden after childbirth:

1. Things that have a lowering effect on the constitution such as fruits and vegetables.
2. Things that have a heating effect on the blood such as the skate, the Prickly Fish, and *ikan sembiling*, a fish that has poisonous spines on both sides and back.
3. Things that have an irritating effect on the skin, such as *ikan tenggiri*, shellfish, and eggplant.

4. Things that are supposed to cause faintness, such as gourds and cucumbers.

5. Sugar, chilies, and coconuts.

Some modern commentators add to this list "foods that contain wind" (Chen 1973:201, 1974—1975:347; McArthur 1962:27), a category unknown to the residents of Merchang. When I asked them which foods carried wind, they were at a loss to understand what the expression meant. After some thought, several volunteered that perhaps it referred to foods that make one flatulent.

According to many sources, notably Wilson (1973) and Chen (1973, 1974—1975), so many foods are forbidden that "in practice the resulting diet usually consists of rice, pepper, chilies, dried or salted fish and coffee." Millis (1958) notes that postparturient Malay women avoid shellfish and "toxic" (bisa) fish which are important sources of protein in the normal diet. Siti Hasmah (1968) writes that the postpartum diet is restricted to only one plate of rice with a small piece of salted fish, black pepper, and only one glass of water a day. Kuah even takes away the bit of fish from the hypothetical postpartum diet. He claims that the postparturient mother's food "consists of a plate of rice with salt and pepper only" (Kuah 1972:82). Although they do not agree on the details of the diet, they do agree that it is practiced universally among rural Malays, except in those cases where modernization or individual rebelliousness has caused women to flout the rules (see, e.g., Wilson 1970:282). "These food taboos have been handed down from one generation to another," says Siti Hasmah. "The reasons for these taboos have long been forgotten but nevertheless they are religiously followed. There is medical evidence to show that these food taboos are harmful to health . . ." (Siti Hasmah 1968:11). According to Siti Hasmah, postpartum food restrictions, kept up for forty days, lead to polyneuritis of thiamine deficiency.

Wilson believes that the Malay postpartum diet, based upon

"ancient superstitions and long-standing custom," (Wilson 1973:267) puts new mothers at risk for anemia. Were the normal diet so unbalanced as we have been led to believe, and the diet during pregnancy so protein-deficient because of superstitious beliefs, it would be amazing if a postpartum diet such as has been described had such relatively mild effects. One might wonder, rather, how one generation could have survived to hand these taboos down to the next.

The authorities agree, as well, that fluids are restricted during the postpartum period, but only a few specify the restrictions. Chen (1974—1975:346) says a new mother is allowed two or three glasses (400—600 ml) of water a day. Siti Hasmah (1968:10) says one glass a day. Millis (1958:141) states that "fluids are also restricted and although only a few women avoided tea or coffee, cold water was not drunk. Fluid restriction has an adverse effect on milk production." This, of course, is true, and is recognized as such by bidan kampung in Merchang, who believe that the supply of breast milk will suffer from insufficient fluid intake. There is no statistical basis for stating that failure of lactation is, in fact, widespread among Malay women. McArthur (1962), working on the west coast, found very little evidence to support the theory that postpartum practices were causing failure of lactation. In my area on the east coast, I questioned 131 women about their experiences nursing their children. One hundred and three had nursed their babies without bottle supplements for periods ranging from one to over three years, twenty-four mixed nursing with bottle feeding, primarily for the purpose of returning to work, and only four had completely given up breast-feeding in favor of bottle-feeding during the early months of the infant's life. One of the four said that her baby threw up when given the breast, and the other three claimed they were not producing enough milk, causing their babies to cry. How can these statistics be explained if fluids are restricted as drastically as has been reported?

The answer lies within an area discussed in connection with the consumption of vegetables in chapter 2. Sayur, the word for vegetables in standard Malay, is not an all-inclusive term in country Malay. Asking people how much sayur they eat will therefore not provide the data investigators are seeking, and may lead them into believing that the answers they get do in fact represent the truth in terms of their own categories. The same holds true for fluid intake. Millis says that "cold water was not drunk" (1958: 141), but this is not a restriction of all fluids. As the postpartum period is considered an abnormally "cold" time, one would expect cold water to be restricted, as well as tea, a "cold" drink even when served at boiling temperatures. Warm water, coffee, milk, and root medicines are quite another matter. Bidan kampung in Merchang recommend that new mothers drink at least three glasses of akar kayu or sepang kederang a day, three glasses of milk (actually one or two tablespoons of condensed milk dissolved in coffee or hot water), and as much coffee and warm water as they please.

Many normally edible fish are avoided during life crises such as the postpartum period, the postcircumcision period, and certain disease states. The fish that are allowed, however, are the most common and least expensive species, and also among the fattiest, which is interesting in view of the restriction of fried foods during these times. Although at first glance the number of prohibited species seems to promise severe dietary restrictions, in practice there is no reason why the amount of animal protein in the diet should diminish.

It is true that, since the humoral system followed by Malays favors hot over cold foods for postparturient women, some items may disappear temporarily from a new mother's diet. The richness of ambiguity and variability of interpretation of Malay systems of food avoidance, at the practical level, do not allow us the liberty of formulating a simple cause and effect relationship between traditional food beliefs and nutritional health. Without doing damage to their ideological integrity, women who think themselves to be strictly following postpartum dietary restrictions eat as much as they want of rice, fish (both fresh and dried), cassava, breads, cakes and crackers, chilies and spices, many types of banana, durian and rambutan fruits, and milk and eggs. Eggs are eaten every day of the postpartum period, mixed with honey, black pepper, and yeast (all very "hot" foods) by women whose families can afford this luxurious medicine. The wealthiest women also add beef to their postpartum diets.

Much of the variation in adherence to traditional postpartum restrictions, as codified in the literature, exhibited by the women of Merchang is based on a theory of experimentation. Village midwives advise their patients to try a wide variety of foods after the delivery of their first baby, starting with "hot," adding seder-hana (neither "hot" nor "cold"), and, if no adverse reactions develop, finally including "cold" foods in their diet. If new mothers experience no bad effects during their first postpartum period, they may then eat a full diet after each subsequent delivery. Women who experience heavy or lengthy discharge of lochia, stomachache, or any tendency to hemorrhage will be much more cautious about what they eat following future pregnancies. Whether a woman restricts her diet for the full forty days (or even, in a few cases, 100 days), for some portion of the forty days, or not at all, is therefore a function of the individual's measure of caution or bravery and her experiences following delivery of her first child. Some women feel it is the better part of valor to restrict their diets even after the first baby, rather than risk any possible problems.

A variation on this theme has been reported in West Java (Freedman 1954:33). During the first few days following child-birth, before the umbilical stump has fallen off, the mother can eat anything without restriction, but after it falls off she is restricted to the specific foods she has eaten before it fell. Her

[187]

husband goes to the market as soon as the baby is born, to buy every kind of food she would like and they can afford, so as not to restrict her diet later on.

I discovered still another variation when I worked with Puerto Rican mothers in New York City, who also subscribe to humoral theories. Although citrus fruits are usually avoided during menstruation, if a girl has been given some during her first menstrual period she may safely eat them thereafter.

Although deviations from the forty day restricted diet have been presented in the literature as arising from modernization (Whyte 1974:64), exposure to scientific medicine (Chen 1975: 130), or individual flouting of the conventions (Wilson 1970:282), this did not seem to be the case in Merchang. Women in their sixties and older reported the same variation of adherence to postpartum restrictions as is now found among younger women. The bidan kampung, who ranged in age from their fifties to seventies, said that their mothers, who had been midwives before them, had given the same advice to their patients. Of 145 women I interviewed, 39 percent reported that they restricted their diets for the full 40 days, and another 1 percent for 100 days. Twenty-one percent never restricted their diets, another 19 percent did so for a week or less, and the remaining 19 percent for two to three weeks (see table 12). In other words, in this subdistrict, considered very traditional by health authorities, where bomoh and bidan kampung were in great demand, 60 percent of the women were not adhering to the restricted diet for the period specified in the literature. Rather than illustrating wholesale flouting of the conventions, this demonstrates the built-in flexibility of Malay ideology and the existence of rules to break rules previously noted in chapter 3.

The pantang is for the mother's, not her baby's, sake. Food restrictions continue for only a short time relative to the total time of lactation. The mother of a stillborn baby is just as likely to restrict her diet as the mother of a live child.

TABLE 12
OBSERVANCE OF *Pantang*
(postpartum food restrictions)

Duration of observance	% of total	No.
3 days	12	(17)
1 week	8	(11)
2 weeks	9	(13)
3 weeks	10	(15)
40 days	39	(57)
100 days	1	(2)
never	21	(30)

N = 145

OBJECTIVE CRITERIA FOR MEASURING HEALTH CONSEQUENCES OF THE *PANTANG*

In view of the seriousness of claims that postpartum food taboos are a major cause of ill health among Malay mothers, it is important to investigate the basis for such statements. The assumption of a cause and effect relationship between tradition and malnutrition has been based, in good measure, on Wilson's research. As her formulation has been cited in at least three articles by herself and two by Chen, and has been accepted as proven fact by editors of anthropology textbooks (Foster and Anderson 1978:273; McElroy and Townsend 1979:241), it is vital to go to her sources to examine the validity of her assumptions.

Wilson (1973) arrived at a hypothetical (deficient) postpartum diet through observation of two women's meals during the course of a single day each, and interviews with a number of other women. A hypothetical diet can at best, present the norm but cannot suggest the range. Her claim that the Malay postpartum diet is inimical to women's health is based, as well, on the evidence of blood tests. The tests she cites, however, do not support these

[189]

assumptions. The blood samples in question were taken from only two new mothers (Wilson et al. 1970:821). Both were folic acid-deficient and one was also iron-deficient. Both had normal serum vitamin A levels, but one was low in carotene. Since blood carotene levels are no longer considered indicative of vitamin A status, this latter finding must be interpreted in terms of satisfactory nutrition rather than the reverse (Dr. John Smith, Columbia College of Physicians and Surgeons, personal communication, 1981). Neither ecological conditions, economic capabilities, nor even individual health problems of these two mothers are discussed, since these considerations apparently pale in the light of ideology. Attitudes toward food are presented as the most important determinant of nutritional status.

Subsequent authors have used this sparse and incomplete data as the basis for such statements as: "It has been found that such a diet results in low serum levels for folic acid, carotene and iron" (Chen 1974–1975:347). Basing authoritative statements about the health of Malay mothers in general on evidence derived from two women in one community is hardly justified, but the problem goes even deeper. Since blood samples were taken only once from each of these women at the close of the postpartum period, there is no baseline available which could tell us whether they had been in an equivocal state during their pregnancies, whether their nutritional status had remained the same during the puerperium, had deteriorated, or even had improved. When these questions are considered, a more complex picture emerges.

In order to assess the effects of postpartum diet on maternal health, I obtained blood samples and dietary information from women at strategic points during their pregnancies and after they completed the puerperium. The number of the subjects was limited to eight, because the Institute for Medical Research, which was responsible for most of the serum nutrient analyses, considered it unfeasible to commit their limited time and personnel to a project on a larger scale. A complete set of data for each

[190]

woman took an average of eight months to obtain, since it was important to take the first sample during the first trimester, before the increase in blood volume changed the values significantly, and the last sample had to be collected immediately after forty days had elapsed since the delivery. A specimen was also collected during the third trimester. Monitoring subjects for such long periods meant that a considerable investment in time was lost whenever a subject moved away from the area or dropped out of the study as a result of miscarriage, and a replacement had to be found.

Some values are missing, as there were problems connected with transporting blood from Merchang to Kuala Lumpur, some 200 miles away, but I was able to get a complete, or almost complete, series for seven women, and partial figures for two others. Although the sample is small, it provides some basis for forming hypotheses about the effects of the postpartum diet, since status at the close of this period can be compared with that of the first and third trimesters of pregnancy. Furthermore, in a largely serendipitous fashion, the seven women for whom I have good sets of dietary and blood analyses represent every spectrum of adherence to the restrictions of the postpartum diet. Two women (Lijah and Wan Zainab) restricted their diets for forty days. Two others (Rohani and Siti Zarah) restricted their diets for twenty days, one (Cik Rohani) did so for two weeks, and two (Khatijah and Gayah) not at all. These women represent, as well, a variety of economic backgrounds, from the wife of a wealthy tobacco dealer (Wan Zainab); to one slightly lower in the economic scale (Lijah), whose husband owned rubber acreage and a monkey trained to pick coconuts off the trees; three who tapped rubber on other people's plantations alongside their husbands (Rohani, Siti Zarah, and Cik Rohani), and one whose husband was a fisherman (Khatijah). I have incomplete, but interesting, data on two women: Asmah, who lived well on the proceeds of a coffeehouse and shop, and Bisah, whose husband had gone to

[191]

seek work in Singapore, leaving her destitute and dependent on charity for her daily food.

Blood samples were tested for hemoglobin and hematrocrit, vitamin A, thiamine, total protein, albumin, and globulin. Of all those tested, only Bisah showed any serious signs of deficiency, and these were present during the first trimester. Her albumin and vitamin A levels were low and her hemoglobin and PCV were deficient. Clearly, her problems were owing to economics rather than tradition. Malay women's diets are not restricted during pregnancy, and this particular woman did not intend to restrict her postpartum diet for ideological reasons, but could not afford to buy many of the foods she would have liked to eat.

All other women showed satisfactory or high levels for all values tested, except thiamine. Three finished their postpartum periods moderately deficient, including one who restricted her diet for forty days, one who restricted hers for twenty days, and one whose restriction lasted two weeks. Curiously, one of those who restricted her diet for the full forty days (Wan Zainab) had been seriously deficient in thiamine at the start of her pregnancy, but had improved considerably by the end of the puerperium. Both of the women who restricted their diets for forty days, and were coincidentally also the two wealthiest, showed a significant rise in hemoglobin at the end of the postpartum period, compared with values during the first trimester. Two others, including one whose *pantang* lasted fourteen days and another who did not observe any restrictions at all, showed smaller rises in hemoglobin, and the remaining three stayed approximately the same in hemoglobin status at the close of the puerperium as they had been during the first trimester. For all other values, a comparison of the values of the sample taken during the first trimester and that taken at the close of the postpartum period shows no discernible difference between those women who restricted their diets for forty days, those who did so for shorter periods, and those who did not do so at all (see table 13).

[192]

TABLE 13
SERUM NUTRIENT ANALYSIS

Name	RBC Trans-ketolase Act.	% TPP effect	PCV %	Hb grs.	Vit. A ug/100	Total protein	Albumin	Globulin	A/G ratio
1. Those who restricted their diets for 40 days postpartum.									
Wan Zainab									
1st trimester	23	48	35	10.2	55	6.4	3.9	2.5	1.5
3d trimester	—	—	30	9.7	89	5.8	3.5	2.3	1.5
Postpartum	36	17	39	13.1	—	6.8	4.6	2.2	2.2
Ljah									
1st trimester	41	Nil	36	10.8	20	6.0	3.6	2.4	1.5
3d trimester	44	Nil	32	10.6	24	6.8	4.1	2.7	1.5
Postpartum	48	24	35	12.4	25	7.4	4.9	2.5	1.9
2. Those who restricted their diets for 20 days postpartum.									
Rohani									
1st trimester	—	—	35	11.0	25	6.0	4.1	1.9	2.1
3d trimester	—	—	37	11.8	20	6.5	2.9	3.6	0.8
Postpartum	—	—	37	11.4	31	8.3	4.5	3.8	1.2
Siti Zarah									
1st trimester	—	—	38	12.5	36	7.2	4.2	3.0	1.4
3d trimester	68	Nil	32	11.2	30	6.1	3.5	2.8	1.2
Postpartum	48	25	43	12.5	43	7.9	4.5	3.4	1.3

TABLE 13 (Continued)
SERUM NUTRIENT ANALYSIS

Name	RBC Trans-ketolase Act.	% TPP effect	PCV %	Hb grs.	Vit. A ug/100	Total protein	Albumin	Globulin	A/G ratio
3. Those who restricted their diets for 14 days postpartum.									
Cik Rohani									
1st trimester	89	Nil	39	12.5	22	6.1	3.8	2.3	1.7
3d trimester	63	Nil	35	11.0	25	6.7	4.1	2.6	1.6
Postpartum	57	18	39	13.1	23	7.2	4.0	3.2	1.3
4. Those who never restricted their diets postpartum.									
Khatijah									
1st trimester	—	—	39	12.8	33	5.8	4.3	1.5	2.9
3rd trimester	—	—	37	12.4	30	6.7	3.5	3.2	1.1
Postpartum	54	5	42	12.8	—	—	—	—	—
Gayah									
1st trimester	43	1	37	11.0	29	6.7	4.1	2.6	1.6
3d trimester	—	—	37	12.4	32	7.3	3.4	3.9	0.9
Postpartum	—	—	32	12.4	30	7.1	4.2	2.9	1.5

5. Those for whom the series is incomplete.

Asmah

1st trimester	—	—	39	12.8	20	6.7	3.5	3.2	1.1
3rd trimester	56	Nil	37	11.0	30	6.7	3.4	3.3	1.0

Bisah

1st trimester	122	Nil	29	8.5	11	6.4	2.5	2.9	1.21

N.B. Gaps represent clotted or otherwise spoiled samples. Samples were taken in three containers and analyzed in two laboratories, so it occasionally happened that the contents of one container was unusable while the others remained unspoiled.

Asmah's pregnancy resulted in a stillbirth. She declined to give a postpartum sample since she suspected that the previous bleedings were implicated in her misfortune. Bisah left the community before I could complete the series.

Nutritional Assessment—guidelines for dieticians (1977) by Ann Grant (privately printed), was used to determine the nutritional implications of laboratory tests on blood.

These blood analyses, while involving a greater number of Malay mothers than had previously been tested (see Wilson et al. 1970), and providing a baseline from which to attempt to judge the health consequences of postpartum food restrictions, still represent a small number of women in a particular ecological setting. It would be premature and highly unwise to generalize from this data other parts of Malaysia, where pre-pregnant health status may be much more precarious, or availability of foods much more limited. It is sufficient, at this point, to say that for this sample of women there is no indication that the postpartum diet led to either anemia or polyneuritis of thiamine deficiency. The data regarding thiamine status are unclear, since levels went down for some women and improved for others who practiced pantang for the full forty days. The data regarding hemoglobin is much clearer. For this sample of women, it would be impossible to implicate postpartum food restrictions as a cause of anemia.

Besides serum nutrient analyses and clinical signs of malnutrition, average birth weights are an important indicator of the nutritional status of the mothers. Average birth weights fall as socioeconomic or nutritional status deteriorates (Hytten and Leitch 1971:311). I collected a random sample of birth weights for fifty children born in Merchang from 1974 through 1976. The average was 3,493 grams. This compares well with mean birth weights for Great Britain. The average birth weight for women under five feet one inch in Aberdeen, Scotland, in 1968 was 3,114 grams (Hytten and Leitch 1971:307). Since very few Malay women exceed the height of five feet one inch, it would seem, judging from their babies' birth weights, that the mother's nutritional status was good.

It is fruitless to attempt any quantitative statements regarding diet without knowing the range as well as the norm. The only method of approaching accuracy in determining the nutritive content of a subject's food intake is to weigh and measure everything that passes her lips. Besides obtaining blood samples, I also collected dietary information during pregnancy and the postpartum period from each woman, for periods ranging from four to fourteen successive days. Analysis of these diets shows an enormous range of values from day to day.

Within a successive five day interval, daily caloric values ranged from 35 percent of the RDA to 96 percent. Protein values ranged from 29 percent to 125 percent, and ascorbic acid from a low of 2 percent to a high of 2,000 percent of the RDA. Similar variations were noted in vitamin A intake. Although many women had a daily intake ranging from 100 to 400 mcg, an occasional day's intake could reach 3840 mcg. In the case of calcium one woman took in 74 mcg one day and 1,178 mcg on another occasion. The spectacular rise in ascorbic acid was due to eating guavas, which grow abundantly in the area. They are not eaten on a daily basis, but people occasionally eat a number of them at a time. The rise in vitamin A intake was caused by a large portion of *cekor manis*, a common wild leafy vegetable. This is the only wild vegetable in the area for which values have been worked out, and there is a strong possibility that similar wild vegetables are equally high in vitamin A content. The increase in calcium was owing to a large amount of shrimp paste (*belacan*). This wide diversity underlines the dangers of relying, as Wilson did, on data derived from one day's meals.

Before discussing these diets in relation to Recommended Dietary Allowances, I would like to point out that RDAs are not requirements, but only recommendations that exceed the needs of most people. There are differences of opinion among nutritionists about the validity of values for requirements and allowances. There is, as well, a paucity of information about requirements for some nutrients. Recommendations of official bodies have tended to reflect both physiological and "social" requirements (those that conform to the current food habits of the population from which they were derived). Both of these

[197]

requirements, which differ from population to population, are frequently used as standards for groups from which they were not derived. Even when average physiological needs can be precisely assessed, it is customary to add an arbitrary allowance for safety (in the case of protein, approximately 30 percent). Individuals vary widely in their requirements, and it would be wrong to conclude, without clinical evidence, that because the diet of an individual woman falls short of the RDA, it is therefore inadequate. It is interesting to note that recommended allowances have become smaller as knowledge has improved (Hytten and Leitch 1971:410, 419).

Using Suggested Daily Dietary Intakes for Peninsular Malaysia (Teong 1975) as a measure, we find that in most respects both the antepartum and postpartum diets of all the women in my sample are low for many nutrients. This cannot be blamed on tradition or ideology, since Malays do not believe in restricting the diets of pregnant women. Surprisingly, the postpartum restricted diet is occasionally higher for some values than the same woman's antepartum diet. For example, Wan Zainab's pantang diet was considerably higher in protein, fat, thiamine, and niacin than her ordinary diet, and Lijah's pantang diet was higher in calories, protein, and thiamine than her diet during pregnancy.[1] This may be due to the relatively high economic status of these women. Although certain items in their diets were restricted, they were able to enhance their diets in a manner congruent with their ideology to more than make up for the lacks.

Comparing the U.S. RDAs with those for peninsular Malaysia, we find that the suggested calorie intake is slightly higher for Malaysian women than for Americans, which is unrealistic since the average weight on which U.S. RDAs are based is 128 pounds, while the average Malay woman's weight is about 100 pounds. The only woman who approached the suggested caloric allowance was Wan Zainab, who appeared considerably overweight, with Lijah running a close second both in caloric intake and excess weight. The other women were well built and not thin, although they were eating considerably less than the suggested allowance.

Other recommended allowances are similar in both tables, with the exception of iron, which is 18 mg for the U.S. and 28 mg for Malaysia. The higher standards for Malaysia are probably meant to offset worm loads. In analyzing only the food intake, we find that none of the women's iron intake came up to even the lower RDA for the U.S. However, if we take into account that all the food was cooked in iron pots, our assessment of dietary iron intake increases considerably—up to two to three times higher for cooked foods—since the iron of the cookware is transferred to the food and ingested (Goodhart and Shils 1973:300).

Low levels of vitamin A intake on any particular day need not be viewed with too much alarm, since we know that most people in Merchang include wild and cultivated green leafy vegetables as part of their diets on some days. The very high amounts of vitamin A found in a portion of cekor manis (4,650 mcg per 100 grams) will ensure that enough vitamin A is stored on the days that this and similar vegetables are consumed to protect people on those days when their vitamin A intake is low.

It is common knowledge that fat-soluble vitamins, such as vitamin A, can be stored in the body. It is less well known that, through tissue saturation, the human adult stores sufficient amounts of vitamin C to carry him through several months of deprivation (Burton 1965:113). Although occasional days show an extremely high intake of ascorbic acid, a number show little or none. There are sources of vitamin C, such as the guava, available year-round, which provide three times the RDA to those who eat just 100 grams. Other fruits, also available throughout the year, have lower but still appreciable yields of ascorbic acid. Seasonal fruits, such as the durian and rambutan, provide 24 and 48 mcg per 100 grams respectively. When they are available, they are eaten in enormous quantities. Since none of my subjects, or other villagers as far as I was aware, suffered from the symptoms of

[199]

ascorbic acid deficiency—petechiae, purpura, and ecchymoses (various forms of internal hemorrhaging which appear as bruise-like spots on the skin), or impared wound healing (and I would have been aware of this since I treated many wounds)—it seems safe to assume that there was sufficient, if irregular, intake of ascorbic acid.

Although niacin intake was generally low, it was much higher than the amount (4.4 niacin equivalents/100 kcal) to which test subjects were limited for up to eighty-seven weeks, with no symptoms of pellagra developing (Horwitt 1956). The body can convert tryptophan, an essential amino acid, into niacin. This capacity becomes more effective during pregnancy (Hytten and Leitch 1971:428). Since fish is high in tryptophan and there is an appreciable amount, as well, in such common dietary items as mustard greens, spinach, and other green leafy vegetables, rice and eggs, it is likely that people in Merchang were getting a significant amount of niacin from tryptophan conversion. This, however, would not appear in the dietary analysis.

Thiamine intake may pose a problem, considering the change, in three subjects, from an unproblematic state in pregnancy to a moderate postpartum deficiency. It is possible that this deficiency was transitory and would disappear with the resumption of a normal diet. It is also possible that, had these women been in a precarious state before and during pregnancy, any further dietary restriction might have increased a preexisting deficiency. The data is clouded, however, by the fact that one subject who restricted her diet for forty days changed from very deficient in thiamine at the start of her pregnancy to almost normal at the close of the puerperium. Her relatively high economic status may be the key to her improved nutritional status. Although Wan Zainab believed herself to be adhering without deviation to postpartum restrictions, she supplemented her diet with beef, eggs, and other foods which many Malay women are unable to afford.

Wan Zainab's comfortable circumstances, which allowed her to have her tradition and eat it, too, contrast vividly with Bisah's poverty, which robbed her diet of essential nutrients in spite of her decision against observing pantang. Although a case might be made for an indictment of poverty, the charge against Malay traditions as the major cause of maternal ill health must be returned with a verdict of "Not guilty."

SUPERNATURAL DANGERS DURING THE PUERPERIUM

The newborn and his mother are vulnerable to attacks from spirits during the postpartum period—he, because his little body is tired after its long journey from the darkness of the womb to the light of day; she, because her body is tired from the exertions of giving birth. The infant's semangat has a precarious hold on its new lodgings; the mother's semangat has been depleted by her labors. Semangat is the body's gate, protecting the home against intruders. When the essential vitality is depleted, the gate loses its integrity and spirits may use the opening to launch an attack.

The hantu most likely to afflict a new mother and her child are the Earth Spirits, who do not confine their activities to infants and their mothers, and the *Hantu Meroyan*, who do. The Earth Genie and his crew are attracted by the sweet smell of the blood of parturition and the lochia of the puerperium. The Hantu Meroyan arises from the afterbirth, the blood, and the amniotic fluid. These incidental products of childbirth, the baby's unsatisfied older siblings, may vent their spleen on both mother and child during the puerperium, and increase their "brother's" illness or misfortunes at other vulnerable times in his life. After the postpartum period, however, this entity is no longer referred to as Hantu Meroyan. It appears during healing ceremonies, using the shaman's lips to complain about the parents' unequal division of their patrimony: The human sibling received his parents' love and property, while the afterbirth had to be contented with a half coconut shell and a scrap of cloth. The placenta is not the baby's

[201]

implacable enemy, however. When he smiles and gurgles with no apparent immediate stimulus, it is because his invisible older brother, the placenta, is playing with him.

The Hantu Meroyan usually gets no opportunity to bother either mother or child because they are protected by the bidan's preliminary lepas. If she neglects the lepas, or performs it badly, the hantu may seize its chance to afflict the nursing couple. Malays arm themselves against such spirit incursions with thorns placed beneath the house and sharp metal objects kept close at hand. The new mother often sleeps with a knife under her pillow. Another knife may be placed under the baby's mattress or near his hanging cradle. Since the Earth Spirits often attack by kicking their victim's big toe, new mothers may tie magically treated cords around their great toes as a kind of spiritual tourniquet. Let the Earth Genie kick her toes as much as he pleases, his noxious influence will not penetrate beyond the cords. A powerful specific against the Hantu Meroyan is a piece of umbrella handle placed in each of the four corners of the fire source under the salaian. The umbrella, symbol of royal rank, is a warning to the spirits that the mother is a subject of the sultan, who has inherited his ancestor King Solomon's dominion over the unseen world.

Occasionally the midwife's spiritual prophylaxis and the family's precautions are not enough to prevent the Hantu Meroyan from interfering with the normal course of the puerperium. An afflicted infant cries incessantly and refuses its mother's breast. An afflicted mother becomes irritable, loses her appetite, finds it hard to sleep, and cries for reasons unknown to herself and her family. She may lose all interest in caring for herself and her child. These, of course, are the symptoms of "postpartum blues," ascribed by some western scientists to the many hormonal changes taking place, by others to unresolved emotional problems, and by still others to a combination of both. Malays believe that women who have been saddened or angered during the postpartum period will be predisposed to *sakit meroyan*. Some women use this belief to exact the kind of considerate or even deferential treatment from their husbands, during the postpartum period, which they might like to have, but wouldn't dare to expect, at other times.

Serious cases of sakit meroyan appear to correspond to postpartum psychosis, a pathological condition for which American doctors recommend extensive psychotherapy. Bomoh treat mild cases of sakit meroyan with incantations, magically treated water, and limes. They may also perform a lepas, on the assumption that the midwife's lepas was inept or insufficient. If the mother's condition does not improve, or if her symptoms are serious, her family may decide to hold a spirit-raising seance (*Main Puteri*) This is usually a treatment of last resort, since it involves a good deal of preparation and expense. The performers of even the most modest Main Puteri include the shaman, his assistant (the *minduk*), a drummer, and a player of the floor cymbals (*cenang*), frequently substituted for by upended pots and a stick. Each of the players must be paid and a ritual meal must be provided for them. Main Peteri can take from one to three nights. The shaman, in trance, first takes on the personae of the inner forces or guardians of the body, his own and those of the patient. He strengthens and restores her semangat. One by one the hantu are persuaded to speak through the shaman's mouth, and to respond to the questioning of the mindok. When it is discovered which hantu are responsible for the patient's sickness, they are threatened, cajoled, or bribed into leaving. The patient is encouraged to go into trance. While in trance she can laugh and cry, sing and dance, and even flirt with the bomoh. She can express the emotions that have been rankling, unexpressed, within her. She emerges from the trance refreshed, greeted by the approval of her friends and relatives who have been watching the ceremony. Their overt show of concern, and the opportunity to express her feelings in an appropriate and unthreatening setting, usually serve to cure the postpartum patient (Laderman 1980). After one

[203]

such session, a new mother who had refused to nurse or even look at her baby was able to smile and gather her baby in her arms. The spell of the Hantu Meroyan was broken.

RELEASE FROM THE POSTPARTUM PERIOD

The ceremony that marks the end of the postpartum period releases the mother from her liminal state and returns her to everyday life within her community. While she is on the threshold, the dietary and other behavioral changes she observes set her apart from normal kampung life. The new mother is not physically segregated from her neighbors and she is not regarded as polluting to others, despite Winstedt's suggestion that she is secluded from men for fear they might suffer contagion from her womanly characteristics (1951:107). Men and women, married and unmarried, fertile and barren, visit the newborn and its mother, who are not obliged to keep their distance or remain in seclusion. Turner (1964:341) observes that those in the liminal state are often symbolically sexless or bisexual. While it is hard to conceive of a woman who has just fulfilled the biological function of her sex as sexless, there is some basis, however, for ascribing symbolic sexlessness to the new Malay mother.

According to tradition, the new mother is barred from engaging in sexual relations until the close of the postpartum period. Some Malay women say that the old and unattractive clothing they wear during the forty days following childbirth has a dual function. It preserves their good clothing from blood stains and smoke damage, and it preserves the wearers from the sexual attentions of their husbands. All too often this tradition is superceded by a stronger cultural rule: a wife disobeys her husband at her own risk. Better to accede to his wishes even three days after delivery (as one of my informants remarked) than face his displeasure and the danger of divorce. "It didn't hurt too much," she said, "and it would have been worse for me if I had refused."

The ceremony that marks the end of the liminal period and releases the new mother from its attendant dangers is known as *rombak dapur*, literally, dismantling the oven and actually, referring to the removal of the salaian. When forty days or so have elapsed, the new father asks the bidan kampung to perform her final services for his wife and child. The ceremony may be an occasion for a large party, or it may be performed privately, with only the immediate family present.

While most people consider it essential to invite the bidan to rombak dapur, some, trying to economize, attempt to do it themselves. If the mother and child continue to be healthy, the amateur lepas may be considered a success. Health problems occurring even years later, however, may be blamed on its insufficiency or ineptitude. My thrifty assistant did not invite the bidan to rombak dapur after his youngest child was born. His wife and baby both developed severe asthmatic conditions. When the baby was close to two years old, a famous visiting bomoh from Kelantan diagnosed their troubles as stemming from a faulty lepas, which he attempted to correct. Besides risking danger, those who do their own lepas may find it difficult to interest the bidan in their wives' future deliveries. In addition to robbing the midwife of her livelihood, they have endangered her health. A bidan who is not released from the dangers of having witnessed the mystery of birth runs the risk of dimmed vision (*carar*).

When the bidan arrives, the keras, kept since the baby's birth, is once more employed as essential ritual equipment. The bidan prepares the other necessary ingredients: neutralizing rice paste (tepung tawar), *pelepas* (double slipknot palm fronds), water, limes, and a chicken or forked stick, depending on the particular midwife's traditions concerning the proper way to rombak dapur. Each bidan plays her own variations on this cultural theme.

Midwives who employ chickens start the ritual by sprinkling rice in the now unlit dapur (fire source for the salaian) to entice the bird to scratch among the cold ashes. When the woman is

[205]

about to be released from the dangers of childbirth, the hantu may seize their final opportunity to rush in and wreak havoc. The chicken, a stand-in for the woman and a symbol of semangat, protects her from their onslaughts. Some midwives substitute a forked stick, which they use to scatter the ashes in the dapur before pitching it out an open window. The stick absorbs the danger of the liminal period and carries it outside the house, leaving the inhabitants safe inside.

Rice paste is sprinkled on the tungku stones, painted on the foreheads of mother, baby, and bidan, and mixed in the bath water. One family that had neglected to prepare rice powder was allowed to substitute talcum powder. The midwife considered its close resemblance to the real thing enough to ensure its efficacy.

The string that had been coiled on top of the keras is now used to release the woman and her child from the postpartum period. In a reenactment of birth and rebirth, the mother and baby pass through the string, the mother passing through three times and her more vulnerable child passing through six times. Mother and baby are bathed with water to which lime juice and rice paste have been added. Water, the universal solvent, washes the dangers of childbirth from the pair and continues the process of symbolic rebirth.

The ritual concludes as the bidan holds up a pelepas and recites a Malay jampi or Arabic prayer, ending with the chanting of "1, 2, 3, 4, 5, 6, 7, you are released!" At these words, the bidan pulls apart the slipknots of the pelepas, graphically releasing the new pair from their long period of vulnerability.

If the baby is a girl, the rombak dapur is used as the occasion of her circumcision. This is a clitorodotomy, or incision of the clitoris, rather than a clitorodectomy, or excision. The infant is held on her mother's or grandmother's lap and her genitals are exposed. The midwife makes a tiny cut with a razor blade or knife. Only a microscopic amount of tissue is removed, not enough to impair the organ's function but sufficient to satisfy tradition.

[206]

Since the baby's diet includes little besides her mother's milk, no food restrictions, such as those imposed on adolescent boys following circumcision, are necessary.

After the bidan helps the family to remove the dapur and salaian and cleans the floor on which they had stood, a communal meal is served to celebrate the incorporation of the pair. The bidan's tasks are over, the new pair has passed safely through the dangers of childbirth, and a new member has joined the community.

· 8 ·

Conceptions and Preconceptions

A careful analysis of childbirth and nutrition in Merchang shows that knowledge of a people's ideology is insufficient to predict their behavior. Ideology provides the basic script, but the actors are not constrained to follow it in detail. They interpret and improvise, often by appealing to rules to break rules. Behavior is meaningful only in context. An actor's world view contains symbols that infuse events with meanings through a dialogue with empirical perceptions—a dialogue replete with insights, delusions, and ambiguities that, in the flow of events that constitutes social life, constantly modify and renew symbol systems. Interchanges between ideology and behavior in any particular culture cannot be understood without a long-term intimate acquaintance with the minutiae of daily existence, the piling up of details that ultimately, miraculously, arrange themselves into complex patterns.

The dynamic relationship of symbol and substance, this lack of congruence between belief and action, has all too often been ignored by investigators of nutritional problems in the Third World. Following the lead of such figures as Jacques May and Derrick Jeliffe, these investigators maintain that ignorance and stubborn devotion to mistaken ideologies are root causes of malnutrition. Western and Western-trained commentators have

[208]

claimed that Malay food ideologies produce bad nutrition, that superstitious beliefs rob the pregnant mother and her family of protein, and that postpartum traditions result in health problems ranging from anemia to madness, or even death. Seen from this perspective, the Malays appear to be the very model of a peasant people whose ignorance of the relationship between food and health, combined with a tenacious clinging to outmoded and maladaptive traditions, is a major cause of ill health. But how rigid and ignorant are these peasants and to what other nutritional ideas are we comparing theirs?

Malays believe that rice is essential for survival and that fish is necessary for strength. Even if we should disagree, it is impossible to ignore the fact that Malays have made a direct connection between food and health. Furthermore, the positive relationship these rural people have made between good diet and good health (rare among traditional peoples, according to Foster and Anderson 1978:272), is far from inaccurate. Rice, representing the bulk of calories in their diet, is indeed essential for survival. Without a sufficient supply of calories, the body, lacking energy to function, cannot survive. Fish, the Malays' principal source of animal protein, is indeed necessary for strength. Without a complete supply of essential amino acids, the body becomes weak and loses its resistance to infection. Judged by the standards of modern nutritional science, Malay food beliefs leave much to be desired. Judged by the same standards, Western nutritional assumptions of the very recent past were also wanting.

We recognize the frequent divergence between stated belief and actual behavior in our culture, and even celebrate our awareness with a common admonition to children: "Do as I say, not as I do." Can we assume that tribal and peasant peoples' thought processes are so much simpler than ours that they translate beliefs directly into action without the intervening steps which we, ourselves, employ for flexibility of interpretation and rationalization of behavior? Such an assumption can only proceed from ethnocentric bias. We cannot allow differences in class, language, folk-ways, lifestyles, or physical appearance to blind us to the fact that the minds of those we study are as rich, complex, and variable as our own. If we do, we run the risk of constructing automatons in place of living human beings, and endowing them with only enough humanity to represent a limiting case—a case that is limited, in fact, only by an impoverished model.

The Malay proverb, "Let the children die, but do not let traditions die" (*Biar mati anak jangan mati adat*), has been cited as an example of the way traditional people cleave to their customs, even to the detriment of their children. Malay proverbs and poetry, however, rarely yield to a literal translation. In the Introduction to the *Dictionary of the Malay Language* (quoted in Brown 1951:x), Clifford and Swettenham wrote:

> Like French [Malay] is essentially a diplomatic language and one admirably adapted for concealing the feelings and cloaking the real thoughts. Not even in French is it possible to be so polite, or so rude, or to say such rude things with every appearance of exaggerated courtesy, as is the case in Malay.

Malay poetry, still composed in the countryside, uses literary and historical allusions to make subtle points. The everyday language of the village can be cryptic to the ears of an outsider in its use of elision and irony, and references to proverbs. When one of a group of farmers remarked to an investigator examining them for breach of land title, "Let the heat be on the fields" (*Biar panas di padang*), the comment was rightly understood to mean that just as the sun's heat beats down with equal fierceness on all parts of an unshaded plain, so should all the offenders in this case be treated equally and none singled out for harsher punishment (Brown 1951:xi). Similarly, the Malay proverb quoted above cannot be understood literally as linking the sacrifice of children to the observance of tradition. As well as alluding to the ephemerality of individual life and the enduring quality of traditions, it is a way of

[210]

emphasizing the value of customs. Just as it is unthinkable to let one's children die, so, too, it is unthinkable to allow traditions to die.

A vulgar literal translation of a peasant people's words is symptomatic of an equally simplistic reading of their culture. A lack of appreciation of their complexities of thought can lead to the error of believing that, unlike ourselves, they follow traditions blindly, come what may. The Malay case, however, belies this assumption.

I have shown that Malays are not slaves of tradition, but interpret and manipulate customs. The customs themselves are not monolithic but allow for flexibility and variation. Malays say, "Everyone's hair is black, but each one's heart is different" (*Rambut sama hitam, hati berlain-lain*). They do not expect conformity or consensus, but rather variations upon a theme.

The range of variation in Malay belief and behavior has often seemed chaotic to outside observers. Winstedt claimed that Malay beliefs have no system or order of their own, but are like a crazy quilt of Hindu and Islamic thought-scraps superimposed on a background of indigenous animism (1951, 1972c). Wilkinson compared Malay culture to "a sort of museum of ancient customs—an ill-kept and ill-designed museum in which no exhibit is dated, labeled or explained" (1908:64). Some more recent observers have described variations in Malay behavior contrary to their expectations as examples of imperfectly learned ideology or individual rebelliousness (Wilson 1970), as the result of modernization (Whyte 1974), or as due to exposure to scientific thought and technology (Chen 1973, 1974–1975, 1975).

Rather than indicating a breakdown in the system, however, this variation is a sign of the system's inherent flexibility. It is not haphazard: it occurs in relation to an underlying structure.

Other scholars of Malay culture have perceived an overall system of order, Cuisinier (1936, 1951) finding a parallelism between the universal macrocosm and the individual microcosm,

[211]

Endicott (1970) discovering relations between spirit and matter, and Kessler (1977) linking Malay magic to political ideology. Firth (1974), while affirming the basic order of Malay beliefs, emphasizes the ways in which pragmatic choices, skepticism, and experimentation serve to vary the behavior of village Malays.

It seems clear that one can hardly arrive at an understanding of behavior without a knowledge of the structure of belief. But such knowledge of ideology can be neither predictive nor retrodictive of behavior unless it includes those subsidiary cultural clauses that may be termed "rules to break rules." These secondary rules allow exceptions to basic ideology without negating its precepts. Malay pregnancy pantang prohibits the killing of animals, however, "rules to break rules" allow the slaughter of certain kinds of animals under particular conditions. Although a cursory reading of this pantang might seem to predict restrictions on the economic activities and dietary intake of the pregnant woman and her family, the rules within rules produce a very different outcome.

Variation in adherence to postpartum pantang is often caused by the existence of subsidiary rules. Although the rule for postpartum food behavior states that the new mother, who is in a "cold" and vulnerable state, should eliminate "cold" and bisa foods from her diet, the subsidiary rule encourages experimentation. New mothers are advised to eat small amounts of many foods following their first delivery. Their experiences during the first postpartum period, interpreted in light of the ideology that gives their experiences meaning, will go far in deciding future behavior.

An internally consistent symbol system is capable of creative individual application in specific circumstances and, indeed, can be reinforced by individual interpretation and manipulation. A knowledge of cultural rules, however, although invaluable in explaining much otherwise incomprehensible behavior, cannot predict individual behavior in all instances. For example, a subsidiary rule of the first puerperium says, "Try everything," but some first-time mothers restrict their diets for fear of the possible consequences of experimentation. On other occasions, beliefs are not implemented by actions that would seem to follow logically, because they cause inconvenience or pain to the actors.

Thus, it is specious to say, for example, that toddler malnutrition among Malays occurs *because* parents believe fish is bad for a young child, or *because* a toddler is believed to be a responsible and independent person (Wolff 1965). Malay parents undoubtedly consider their toddlers to be more responsible, and grant them more independence, than do their American counterparts, but a demand for more fish is more likely to bring the Malay toddler what he wants than to elicit a refusal based on the assumption that he can compete equally with older siblings, or the belief that fish can increase the number of worms in his stomach. "I know I shouldn't give it to him," say the mothers, "but who can stand that crying?"

To what extent are the flexibility and complexity of Malay society, as I have represented them, attributes unique to this people, and to what extent are they reflections of the anthropologist's theoretical bias? An assessment of the validity of any study must include considerations of the investigator's preconceptions as well as those of his subjects. I cannot assume that the Malay case represents a *lusus naturae* in a world typified by people whose rigid ideologies lead them into equally rigid behavior, punctuated only by individual rebellion or modified by acculturation. I believe that our vision of the human condition more closely approaches reality if we conceive of interpretation of ideology and "rules to break rules," modifying behavior, as common features of all cultures which can be found if investigators are prepared to expect them, and to search for the structures upon which variations rest.

[213]

Glossary of Malay Words
Used in the Text

Vowels approximate the Italian pronunciation.
c is pronounced like English *ch*, as in *church*.
k at the end of words represents a glottal stop.
Final *t* is unaspirated.

adat—custom, tradition.
air tawar—magically treated water.
akar kayu—medicine made from roots and herbs.
angin—1. wind.
       2. flatulence.
       3. talent, predeliction.
badan—1. body.
       2. a painful eczemalike skin condition.
badi—an evil principle or destroying influence.
badi mayat—the badi of a human corpse. If a pregnant woman is
    exposed to a corpse, Malays believe that her baby may be born
    with badi mayat, a sickness whose symptoms mimic a corpse's
    appearance, and which usually ends in the baby's early demise.
belacan—shrimp paste.
berlendir—the quality of having lendir (see below).

[215]

bertih—popped rice.

bidan—midwife.

bidan kampung—village midwife; traditional birth attendant.

bisa—toxic; an intensifier of internal physical disharmonies. During the postpartum period, bisa specifically refers to foods which are believed to produce postpartum hemorrhage or digestive disorders.

bomoh—Malay indigenous medical practitioner.

buah—1. fruit.

      2. internal stomach abcesses.

budu—fermented liquified anchovies.

cinabuta—a paid interim husband who briefly marries a woman divorced with three talak (see below), in order to enable the original couple to remarry in accordance with religious law.

dapur—1. stove.

      2. the fire source for the salaian (see below).

daun kayu—wild vegetables.

demam—fever.

demam panas—hot fever.

demam sejuk—cold fever, usually referring to chills, or the cold phase of malaria.

hari jatuh benih—the human fertile period; literally, the day the seeds fall.

hantu—disembodied spirits.

hujan panas—a sunshower; literally, hot rain.

iddah—period during which widows and divorcees may not remarry.

ikan—fish.

ilmu—knowledge; frequently, magical knowledge.

jampi—incantations.

jin—genie.

Jin Tanah—the Earth Spirit.

jinggi—see badi.

kampung—village, hamlet.

kati—625 grams.

kenduri—communal feast.

keras—ritual object consisting of a plate of raw rice, some coins, a husked coconut, and a length of raw cord looped atop the coconut.

khalwat—close proximity, in a secluded place, of a Muslim woman and a man to whom she is not married—a civil as well as religious crime.

kuwung—see badi.

lauk—side dish eaten with rice.

lekat kenan—birth defect believed to be caused by prenatal influence.

lendir—phlegm in humoral terminology; slime. Used to describe mucus, egg whites, semen, viscous matter in plants, lymph.

lenggang perut—literally, rocking the abdomen. Refers to the ceremony performed for primigravidae during the seventh month of pregnancy.

lepas—to release; a ritual action used to take people out of a state of danger.

Main Puteri—shamanistic performance, usually used for healing and exorcising.

meroyan—postpartum depression or psychosis.

minduk—a bomoh who takes the part of interlocutor in the Main Puteri (see above).

mukim—subdistrict; parish.

musim—season.

musim banjir—season of floods (monsoon).

musim kemarau—dry season.

musim sejuk—cold season (monsoon).

nasi—cooked rice.

nasi semangat—glutinous rice cooked in coconut cream and colored yellow with turmeric, served at weddings, circum-cisions, and other ritual occasions.

nyawa—breath of life.

padi—unhusked rice.
panas—hot, thermally or humorally.
panas hati—hot-tempered.
pandai—1. expert, clever.
      2. developmentally ready.
pantang—prohibited by custom, or on medical grounds.
pelepas—ritual object consisting of two strips of palm frond tied together in a double slipknot, used to release people from a state of danger.
pelesit—a familiar spirit associated with women.
penawar—antidote, remedy.
rombak dapur—dismantling the "roasting bed," the ceremony that releases the new mother from the postpartum period.
ruh—soul.
sakit—1. illness.
      2. pain.
sakit angin—Malay illness category similar to the Western category of psychosomatic ailments.
salaian—"roasting bed."
sambang—an illness of neonates believed by Malays to be caused by the infant's having been born with the umbilical cord looped around its neck.
sayang—1. love, affection.
      2. pity.
      3. of a fetus, so firmly ensconsed in the womb that it is impossible to dislodge either accidentally or deliberately.
sayur—1. in standard Malay, vegetables.
      2. in east coast dialect, vegetables cooked sayur style, i.e., with fish, coconut milk, and spices.
sederhana—1. medium, average, the proper mean.
      2. neutral, in a humoral sense.
sejuk—cold, thermally or humorally.
semangat—life force, embodied spirit.

sesuai—harmonious.

sipat—outward characteristics.

talak—formula of divorce.

tepung tawar—neutralizing rice paste used in rituals.

terima—to receive, used for receiving the mantle of a bidan or bomoh.

tungku—heated stone wrapped in cloth and placed on the abdomen of a woman in the puerperium.

ubat—medicine.

ulam—raw vegetables eaten as salad.

zat—1. essence of food, nutritive value.

2. hidden esoteric characteristics or aspects.

Appendix 1

EDIBLE WILD PLANTS CONSUMED IN MERCHANG

Vegetables
1. Balek adab (Fam. Rubiaceae, possibly Mussaenda sp.)
2. Bayam ngang (Fam. Compositae).
3. Bayam peraksi (Fam. Compositae).
4. Binan setukar (Decaspermum frutenscens Fam. Myrtaceae).
5. Cekor manis (Sauropus androgynus).
6. Deber lembu (Fam. Compositae).
7. Gajah nangis (Saraca sp. Fam. Leguminosae).
8. Gelam tikus (Eugenia sp.).
9. Gucil (Antisdesma ghaesembilla Fam. Euphorbiaceae).
10. Jeneris (Connarus ellipticus).
11. Kayu kelat (Eugenia sp. Mytacaea).
12. Keladi agak (Monochoria vaginalis Fam. Pontederiacerae).
13. Kerkoh batu (Myrica esculenta Fam. Myricaceae).
14. Kulat batu (Lentinus sajor-caju).
15. Kulat sisir (Schizophyllum).
16. Kulat telinga tikus (Auricularia auriculae-judae).
17. Lapeng budak (Clerodendron sp. Fam. Verbenaceae).
18. Leban (Vitex pubescens Fam. Verbenaceae).

[221]

19. Lidah katung (unidentified).
20. Paku hijau (Ceropteris).
21. Paku merah (Nephrodium).
22. Paku piah (Cycus cfr. rumphii Fam. Cycadaceae).
23. Pinan keroh (Cnestis palala Fam. Connaraceae).
24. Pokok kuat (Ploiarium alterniforium Melch. Fam. Myricaceae).
25. Pucuk midin (Stenochlaena palustris).
26. Putak (Barringtonia sp. Fam. Lecythidaceae).
27. Rebung buluh (Bambusa: bamboo shoots).
28. Sawa bubu (Possibly Thizophoraceae or Rubiaceae).
29. Sepit (Either Sesuvium portulacastrium or Portulaca oleraceae).
30. Serai kayu (unidentified).
31. Serian (Cissus sp. Fam. Vitaceae).
32. Sisek puyu (Carallia).
33. Sugidama (Possibly Guioa Fam. Sapindaceae).
34. Terung pipit (Solanum torvum).
35. Tudung periok (Fam. Rubiaceae, probably an Ixora sp.).
36. Ulat bulu (Passiflora foetida).

Edible Palm Cabbages, obtained from both wild and domesticated individuals of the following species:

1. Umbuk bayas (Oncosperma horrida).
2. Umbuk kelapa (Cocos).
3. Umbuk nibung (Oncosperma tigillaria).
4. Umbuk palas (Licuala).
5. Umbuk pinang (Areca).

Fruits

1. Asam gelugor (Garcinia sp.).
2. Buah berangan (Castanopsis sp. Fam. Fagaceae).

3. Buah beruas (Garcinia hombroniana Pierre Fam. Gutti-ferae).
4. Buah berus (Bruguiera parviflora).
5. Buah binan setukar (Decaspermum frutenscens Fam. Myrta-ceae).
6. Buah gelam tikus (Eugenia sp.).
7. Buah gucil (Antisdesma ghaesembilla Fam. Euphorbiaceae).
8. Buah jentik (Baccaurea).
9. Buah jering (Pithecellobium jiringa).
10. Buah kandis (Garcinia sp.).
11. Buah kayu kelat (Eugenia sp. Mytacaea).
12. Buah keduduk (Melastoma malabathricum).
13. Buah kelubi (Zalacca sp.).
14. Buah kemunting (Rhodomyrtus tomentosa).
15. Buah keredas (Pithecellobium microcarpus).
16. Buah kerkoh batu (Myrica esculenta Fam. Myricaceae).
17. Buah mata ayam (Ardisia crispa).
18. Buah mata kucing (Nephelium malaiense).
19. Buah nipah (Nipa fruticans).
20. Buah palas (Licuala sp. Fam. Palmae).
21. Buah petar (Parkia speciosa).
22. Buah rekan (Zalacca sp.).
23. Buah salak (Zalacca sp.).
24. Buah setial (Sendoricum sp.).
25. Buah setol (Sendoricum indicum).
26. Buah sisik puyu (Carallia).
27. Buah terjang (Erioglossum rubiginosum).
28. Buah ulat bulu (Passiflora foetida).
29. Geratak tangga (Castanopsis sp. Fam. Fagaceae).
30. Nyior lemba (Curculigo sp. Fam. Hypoxidaceae).
31. Rambutan gerat, also known as buah pahit (Nephelium mutabile).

N.B. These plants were identified by Professor Benjamin C. Stone of the Department of Botany, University of Malaya. The division into fruits and vegetables was done by my informants in Merchang. *Buah* usually refers to fruit, *umbuk* to palm cabbage, *paku* to ferns, and *kulat* to fungi.

Appendix 2

INCANTATIONS
Incantation for Difficult Births
(Original Malay Version)

Bismillah, aku mulai awal meletakkan rahsia ini. Tabib belum zahir. Nur belum latas dalam kelimun-lah tiada lagi. Kepada masa Nur terjeli dalam ya illahi dan tatkala bumi belum jadi terdengan langit, aras kerusi belum terdiri, loh mapor belum tersurat kala mula, belum ternyata. Syurga neraka belum terbilang pada masa itu-lah. Tabib minta sekun bertambah raksi di surat awal titah mula. Minta turun kepada aku menjadi bomoh, menjadi tabib serta bomoh, serta aku ucap subaha nallah. Mula Nur Din, mula Nur Dan, mula meletak awal menjadi sekelian loh mapor kalam hadis dalil langit bumi. Lalu lahir ucap yang ketiga. Satu ucap jadikan besi, dua ucap jadikan nyawa, tiga ucap jadikan mani, mani terkepuh jadikan buih, buih duduk dalam laut laki nallah. Lama sekelian lama, 70,000 tahun. Pertama Laut Latih, dua Laut Alam, tiga Laut Fikir, empat Laut Akal, lima Laut Jima', enam Laut Letih, tujuh Laut Sabar, lapan Laut Buih. Buihnya bawa di angin, nya sepak di ombak, alun tujuh, gelombang satu. Mana buih nak jatuh? Lalu buih jatuh di tebing bereke. Anak ru muda-muda dalam negeri mas, Raja Bali Pancur Angin.

Maka turun-lah malaikat ambil buih Jibrail itu mengadap pada Nur Muhammad, bawa pada Nur Muhammad. Maka Jibrail pun bertanya pada Nur Muhammad, "Ya tuanku, apa-lah di dalam buih ini? Warnanya molek, empat bangsa, empat warna." Maka berkata Muhammad, "Ya Jibrail, kalau mu nak tahu dalam buih ini, ambil kersani yang keras-keras, belah dua, pecah empat, jurai lima." Maka Jibrail ambil Persani yang keras-keras, belah dua, pecah empat, jurai lima. Li terjeli dua terdua, kakak bernama Abang Haji Mula, adik bernama Siti Putih Kebaya Bunga. Mulah sungguh benih yang asal, angin yang berusul.

Maka Jibrail pun di tanai pula empat puluh hari, Nur Tit namanya. Maka Jibrail pun di campak di otak bapak empat puluh hari, nama Nur Allah. Jatuh ke mata, Nur Cahaya, jatuh ke dada, Sertan (Sultan) Jati, pusat alam gembira, jatuh ke ibu kaki, Raja Zakar nama nya. Lalu-lah pula mu, tuan hamba, ucap-lah, tuan hamba, empat puluh kali sehari, empat puluh kali semalam. Lalu mu jatuh pula dalam kandungan bapak. Empat puluh hari di, wadi, mani, manikam. Di itu jadikan tanah, wadi itu jadikan air, mani itu jadikan api, manikam itu jadikan angin. Lalu mu jatuh dalam kandungan bonda. Rahim ibu mu sembilan bulan, sepuluh hari, Satu bulan Noktah nama mu, dua bulan Nur Kun, tiga bulan Nur Leruh, empat bulan Nur Sipat, lima bulan Nur Rahim, enam bulan Abdullah Kohor, tujuh bulan salam ke kanan salam ke kiri. Salam ke kanan, anak laki, salam ke kiri, anak perempuan. Lapan bulan Nur Salin, sembilan bulan tapak bayang bayangan di antara, sepuluh keluar-lah. Mu membawa sipat dua puluh Muhammad. Mu kenal jasat ibu, mu celik mata, mu ucap tiga ucap. Satu ucap mengangkatkan sadar ruh, yang kedua mengucap sadar nyawa, tiga ucap mengangkatakan semangat. Rasa mu rasa biar baik. Mu hisap biar kena dalam semangat lima serta mu limbai tiga limbai. Mu bawa jarum seperti jarum hari berdiri-lah mu dalam akoh lima, puak huruf alif, lam, za, ruh, lullah. Mu bangkit sahabat saudara mu, ya Jibrail, ya Mikail, ya Israfel, ya Israel, ya Ali, ya Omar, ya Osman, ya Abu Bakar, ya Kiraman Katibin.

Appendix 2

Contraceptive Incantation

(Original Malay Version)

Bismillah-hir rahman-nir rahim.
Berlendir putih, berlendir batu,
Berlendir aku nak berhancurkan.
Singgah di bukit, bukit pecah.
Singgah di batu, batu patah.
Singgah di padang, padang hangus.
Singgah di rumput, rumput bubus.
Hei cair, aku hendak cair.
Kalau mu tidak cair
Derhaka mu pada Allah.
Bukan kuasa aku.
Berkat kata la-illaha illa'llah Muhammad-ur rasulullah.

Incantation Recited Over Salt Mixture by
Bidan Kampung

(Original Malay Version)

Bismillah-hir rohman-nir rahim.
Jin Tanah, Jembalang Tanah, aku tahulah asalmu.
Punai kuning, aku nak tanam sama aku.
Jadi lalat.
Hei, aku tahu kerana asalmu.
Mu dengarlah aku pesan,
Kalau mu tak dengar aku pesan, aku sumpah mu dakan dakar.
Terbang, jadi abu angin.
Bukan kuasa aku, dengan kuasa Allah.
Sidi guru, sidi aku, sidi guru, sidi berkat kata
La-illaha illa'llah Muhammad-ur rasulullah.
Qul huwallahu ahad. Allahussanad. Lam yalid walam yulad
Walam yakul lahu kufuwan ahad.

Appendix 3

FISH

The numbers in parentheses following the names of *bisa* fish refer to the following reasons given for placing the fish in this category:

1. They have thick skin but thin scales.
2. They have thin skin but thick scales.
3. They are bottom feeders.
4. They eat annelid worms with bristles that cause irritant wounds, jellyfish, or other organisms known to be poisonous to people.
5. They have small sharp bones which are difficult to remove.
6. They are slimy (*berlendir*).
7. They have poisonous spines.
8. They have sharp but not poisonous spines.
9. They have larger scales than would be normal for their size.
10. They have spots.
11. Some people use color as a criterion: red and sometimes yellow.

Appendix 3

"Safe" Fish

(Words in italics after hyphens are the Latin scientific names.)

Seafish

Usual fish eaten after childbirth in Merchang

Celek-Megalaspis cordyla—trevally.
Gelama-Sciaenidae—jewfish.
Gerepoh-Caranx spp.—trevally, horse mackerel, kingfish.
Kembong-Rastrelliger kanagurta—mackerel.
Selar pucat-Selar megalaspis—scad.
Selayang-Decapterus russellii—scad.

Less common, but some people say these are "safe."

Bagat-Caranx ignoblis—horse mackerel, kingfish. (11)
Cermin-Caranx carangus—horse mackerel, trevally.
Cupok (local name). (11)
Gerong-Caranx speciosus—golden trevally. (11)
Kaci-Pectorhyncus pictus—sweetlip.
Keras ekor-Megalaspis cordyla—trevally.
Layur-Trichiurus spp.—ribbonfish. (6)
Lemok-Lactarius lactarius—white fish.
Merah-Lutianus spp.—red snappers. (11)
Petek-Ambassis—sea perch.
Repoh (local name). (6)
Tambong-Clupea spp.—sardine. (6)
Tudung tempayan-Platacidae—batfishes.

Those who avoid the fish mentioned above which have no numbers in parentheses following their names do so because they are uncommon species and therefore they deem it wiser not to eat them.

[229]

Appendix 3

Estuary Fish

Some people say only *ikan gerepoh* is safe and all others are bisa, since they eat mud (bottom feeders). Other people add:

Anding-Mugil borneensis—mullet.

Swamp Fish

Aruan-Rachycentron candus—black kingfish, cobia.
Pelata-Caranx spp.—scad.

Some people add:

Anak seluan-Rasbora—carp.
Belut-Monopterus—swamp eel.
Bujok-Opiocephalus—murrel.

Bisa Fish

Sea Fish

Anak midin (local name). (5, 6)
Aruan tasek-Rachycentron canadus—black kingfish, cobia. (1, 4)
Ayer-Cermo sibi—albacore. (1, also causes itching)
Barat-barat-Ballisteodei—filefish, triggerfish, leatherjacket, tripod fish. (3)
Bawal-Stromateidae—pomfret. (1, 3)
Bayan-Labridae—wrasses, rainbowfishes.
     Callyodontidae—parrotfishes. (2, 9)
Bilis-Stolephorus indicus—anchovy. (5)
Bulan-Megalops cyprinoides—tarpon. (5, sharp scales)
Celek mata-Pomadasys maculatus—grunter. (2, 3, 7)
Conor-Saurus myops, Saurus tumbil—lizardfish. (4, 6)
Delah-Caesio erythrogaster—fusilier, sea bream. (6, 8)
Dengkis-Siganidae—rabbitfish. (7)
Duri-Tachysuridae—catfish. (6, 8)

Gerut-Pomadasys hasta—grunter. (2, 8)

Golok-Coryphaena hippurus—dolphin. (1)

Jebong-Abalistes stellaris—triggerfish. (1, 3)

Kapas-Gerres abbreviatus—silver-biddy. (6)

Kembasi (local name). (5, 6)

Kerisi-Nemipterus hexodon—Threadfin, bream. (3, 11)

Kerong-kerong-Therapondiae—perch, grunters.

          Plectorhyncus cuvieri—sweetlips. (2, 8)

Kikit (local name). (3, 6)

Kurau-Polynemus indicus—threadfin. (10)

Kurau janggut-Polynemus tetradactylus—threadfin. (10)

Kurau pipit-P. heptadactylus—threadfin. (10)

Nipis-Opisthopterus tartoor—longfinned herring. (5)

Parang-parang-Chirocentrus dorab—wolf herring. (5)

Pari-Order *Rajae*—Rays, skates. (6, venomous tail)

Pisang-pisang-Caesio caerulaureus—fusilier.

          Albula vulpes—bonefish. (3, 5, 6)

          Chanos chanos—milkfish.

          Elegantis bipinnulatus—rainbow runner.

Pucok rebong-Clupeoides venulosus—sardine. (6, 10)

Pulutan-Tachysurus spp.—shad. (6, 8)

Remong-Lutianus lineolatus—gold-striped snapper. (5, 6, 11)

Rokok-Pomadsys maculatus—grunter. (6, 8)

Sabelah-Order *Pleuronectiformes*—flatfishes. (1, 6)

Songsong harus-Selar malam—scad. (1, 6)

Talang-Chorineumus spp.—leatherskin. (10)

Tengiri-Scomeromorus spp.—spanish mackerel. (4)

Tiram-Clupea kanagurta—shad. (6)

Togok-Psettodes crumei—halibut. (1, 6)

Estuary Fish

Bayan (see sea fish).

Dukan (local name). (6, 7)

Kakap-Lates calcarifer—cock-up. (10)
Kakap merah-Lutianus argentimaculatus—snapper. (11)
Kekek-Equula (no English name). (6, 8)
Sebokoh-Pomadasys maculatus—grunter. (8)
Sebokok-Ichthyoscopus lebeck—stargazer. (5)
Sembilang-Plotosus canius—catfish eel. (7)
Tanda-Lutianus spp.—snapper. (10)

Swamp Fish

Anak kepala putih (local name). (6, 10)
Anak sekaring (local name)—like Siamese fighting fish, but black.
Anak sepilah-Betta splendens—Siamese fighting fish. (11, also because they are vicious)
Keli-Clarias, Gronovius—catfish. (6, 7)
Kepal-Abudefduf—demoiselle. (8)
Puyu-Anabas scandens—climbing perch. (8)
Selat (local name). (5)
Sepat-Pempheris molucca—sweeper. (5)

Identification of fish done with the assistance of the Bureau of Fisheries, Penang.

Appendix 4

DIETARY ANALYSES

DIETARY ANALYSES

Name	Time	Day	Cal.	Prot.	Fat	CHO	Ca	Fe¹	A	B₁	B₂	Niac.	C
Wan Zainab bt. Cik Mat	Before Fasting	1	2073	42	30	417	248	11. 3	143	.6	.34	2.07	135
	Month²	2	2025	44.6	50.3	366.3	217	21.4	80.6	.65	.14	2.47	241
	Antepartum	Avg	2049	43.3	40.15	392	232.5	16.3	111.8	.62	.24	2.27	188
	Fasting month	1	757	18.6	10	137	103	12.4	163.5	.22	.26	3.46	34.4
	Antepartum	2	1314	20.8	59	134	137	4.8	43	.28	.27	3.1	7
		3	1355	37	35.6	264	521	4.7	282	.41	.73	5.85	35.3
		Avg	1142	25.5	34.9	178.3	253.7	7.3	162.8	.30	1.26	12.4	25.6
	Postpartum	1	2125	62	56	325	198	8.5	140	.43	.75	12.8	0
		2	1749	64	46	266	66.5	8.4	70	.35	.52	10.9	0
		3	2328	91	59	350	38	5.9	229	.68	.87	13.3	0
		Avg	2067	72.	54	313	100	7.6	146	.48	.46	12.3	0
Siti Zarah	Antepartum	1	1942	98	53.6	267	590	16.5	940	1.37	.43	31	23
		2	2324	73.1	82.8	304.2	472.5	28.1	1162	.88	.36	21	38.4
		3	796	30	118.3	117.5	623	10.9	203.5	.13	.26	6.41	23.5
		4	878	20	8.6	180	240	3	419	.16	.16	2.2	115
		Avg	1485	55.3	66	217.2	481.4	14.6	681	.63	.3	15.2	50
	Postpartum	1	1167	38.4	49.5	76.5	50	2.45	60	.12	.19	4.8	0
		2	1007	30.4	17	182	28.8	1.96	40	.15	.13	3.2	0
		3	1629	39.4	47	255	46.5	3.0	40	.16	.13	3.2	0
		Avg	1267.7	36.06	37.8	171.2	41.8	2.47	46.7	.14	.15	3.7	0

Subject	Period	No.											
Bisah Bt. Ismail	Antepartum	1	1498	40	41.5	241	281	5.4	3840	.32	.34	4.5	87
		2	1207	40	29	200	137	3.6	244	.35	.39	6.08	63
		Avg	1352	40	35	220	209	4.5	2042	.33	.36	5.2	75
	Postpartum	1	763	23	28	102	34	1.68	48	.22	1.34	4.5	0
		2	970	36.5	17.3	171	38	2.26	60	.21	.20	5.22	0
		Avg	866	30	22	136	36	1.97	54	.21	.77	4.8	0
Lijah Bt. Yusof	Antepartum	1	1135	30.7	23	198	113	8.3	86	.51	.35	11.1	1088
		2	2075	44	26	429	63.3	8.1	23	.54	.32	6.45	74.7
		3	2169	63	103	426	112	9.5	16	.60	.10	1.4	3.3
		Avg	1793	45.9	50.66	351	96.1	8.63	42	.55	.25	6.31	62.3
	Postpartum	1	2151	37.6	80	319	32	3.8	32	.46	.06	2.6	0
		2	1626	63	6	368	97.4	8	56	.52	.49	2.6	0
		3	1874	48.6	15.7	460	80	11.4	25	.8	.17	2.3	1
		Avg	1883	49.7	33.9	382.3	69.8	7.7	38	.59	.24	2.5	.33
Che Asmah bt. Che Mat	Fasting month	1	1975	66	63.94	271	416.3	9.44	935	.99	.95	7.33	37
	Antepartum	2	2625	64.3	60.20	455	345.3	1.58	341	1.47	.78	9.16	52
		3	2017	72.4	42.80	324	386.5	16.3	560	.39	.45	16.6	40
		Avg	2206	66.20	55.64	350	382.7	11.1	612	.95	.72	11.03	43
	After Fasting Month	1	3242	88.2	129.8	431.5	468.0	7.42	180	.53	.83	10.4	0
		2	2258	75.3	87.0	296.5	245.3	7.50	142.2	.46	.60	10.25	30

[1] Iron values are for food intake only. No allowance has been made in this analysis for dietary iron supplied by cooking in iron pots.
[2] Muslims fast from sunrise to sunset during the month of Ramadan.

Name	Time	Day	Cal.	Prot.	Fat	CHO	Ca	Fe[1]	A	B_1	B_2	Niac.	C
	Antepartum	3	2529	81.8	78.8	339.0	483.5	19.7	577	.28	.42	8.9	40
		Avg	2676	81.76	98.53	355.66	398.93	11.54	299.73	.42	.61	9.85	23.3
	Postpartum	1	2329	58.7	88.7	316.2	254.2	14.13	183	.64	1.115	9.2	94
		2	1406	45.7	35.5	202.65	200.8	5.84	73.5	.226	.793	3.1	0
		3	1444	42.3	36.6	237.4	225.2	5.77	98	.20	.44	5.13	0
		Avg	1726.3	48.9	53.6	252	227	8.58	118	.35	.78	5.81	31.3
Gayah Bt Hassan	Antepartum	1	1275	75	32	152	1178	13.9	150	.35	.39	9.6	23
		2	1405	48.7	40.5	215	256	6.2	2634	.48	.65	8.74	103
		3	2507	118	62.1	359	410	20.3	2102	.86	4.04	14.6	101
		Avg	1729	80.6	44.9	242	615	13.5	1629	.56	1.7	11	75.6
	Postpartum	1	1068	34	7	221	46	3.7	0	.48	.17	5.2	0
		2	804	21	23	127	399	3.3	1355	.2	.43	1.86	37
	week 2	Avg	936	27.5	32	174	222	3.5	677	.34	2.6	3.5	18
	week 3	1	932	33	37	112	44	6	71	.65	.33	7.6	12
		2	1119	28.6	30	183	104	4	230	.31	.38	6.3	90

	Avg	1	33	147	74	5	301	.48	.35	7	51
Avg	1025	31	33	147	74	5	301	.48	.35	7	51
week 5 — 1	763	28	52	222	101	2.1	413	.16	.25	3.7	11
Antepartum 1	2071	42.2	25	444	265	6.4	438	.71	.27	1.7	71
2	337	7.2	3.9	71.5	34	.35	120	.11	.11	1.74	24
3	721	11.6	21	83	150.5	1.73	104	.18	.2	.8	136
Avg	1043	20.3	16.6	200	183	2.8	221	.33	.2	1.4	77
Postpartum 1	1605	56	15.75	309	704	9.05	60	.25	.27	7.5	0
2	1713	63	44.1	342	1018	10.8	498	.37	.43	9.5	36.3
3	1173	40	9.5	224	838	6.7	1056	.24	.39	5.6	216
Avg	1497	53	23.1	292	853	8.9	538	.29	.36	7.5	22

Rohani bt. Suleiman

Notes

1: INTRODUCTION

1. Foods may be restricted or avoided for many reasons other than supernatural sanctions. Although food restrictions are often termed *taboos* (e.g., Wilson 1973), care must be taken to distinguish among these conceptual categories.

2. My description of Merchang refers to conditions during 1975 to 1977. Many important changes have already occurred since that time. It should also be noted that beliefs and practices, as well as environmental and economic conditions, cannot be expected to remain constant throughout Peninsular Malaysia but may vary from state to state, and even within any given state, in certain particulars.

2: FOOD: BELIEF AND BEHAVIOR

1. A list of wild plants eaten in Merchang will be found in Appendix 1.

2. I was unprepared for this extensive use of wild products. In a careful study of the literature, Dunn (1975:95) could find no references to forest collecting by Malays. Wilson (1970:139) mentions the occasional use of wild plants as "poverty" foods.

3. Malays have similar beliefs, which will be discussed in depth in the following chapter.

3: THE MALAY HUMORAL SYSTEM

1. The Chinese system, as reported by Anderson (1980) is, in fact, similar in many details to that of the Malays.

[239]

2. The term *hospital-based medicine* first came to my attention when it was used by Rena Gropper in the late 1960s.

3. For example, in a discussion of the humors in the first book of the Hippocratic corpus, *On Ancient Medicine*, it is stressed that each individual must be considered as a separate case since humors do not exist in the same proportions in everybody (Adams 1886, I:143—144).

4. A feature that is assumed to be present unless otherwise specified is called *unmarked*; if it needs to be specified it is *marked*.

5. It is curious to note that recent thermographic studies reveal that skin temperature of painful areas can be 2 to 6 degrees lower than normal. "The lower temperature of painful areas is a result of constricted blood vessels in the area reducing the flow of warm blood from deep within the body" (Rensberger 1980:C3).

6. Although most cases of hypertension are asymptomatic, some have been associated with throbbing paroxysmal headaches (Holvey and Talbott 1972:1272).

7. I do not mean to imply that Malays recognize hypertension as a biomedically reckoned disease or understand its etiology in scientific terms, an ignorance we share with them. *The Merck Manual of Diagnosis and Therapy* (Holvey and Talbott 1972:465) terms primary hypertension a "disorder of unknown origin" and Stedman's Medical Dictionary (1979:674) says that essential hypertension develops without known cause.

8. Firth (1974) has commented on this vein of skepticism in Malay villages.

9. Although usually glossed as tart or astringent, neither English word is a true translation of kelat in reference to food. The word is not applied to the tartness of lemons, nor does it have the harsh quality we associate with the astringency of alum. It refers, rather, to the taste of certain tropical plants, such as the *Eugenia*, known as *Kelat*, and associated species such as *Anacardia*, for instance, the leaves of the cashew tree.

10. Fat has a high satiety value, since it slows the emptying of the stomach, thus decreasing intestinal motility and delaying the onset of hunger (Burton 1965:76).

11. After ingestion of proteins, the body's heat output is increased by 20 to 30 percent over intake, compared with 5 percent for carbohydrates and fats (Burton 1965:25). This specific dynamic action of protein may contribute to subjective feelings of internal heat claimed by Malays to follow meals featuring "hot" foods.

12. Many American doctors and nutritionists recommend moderate

reduction of animal proteins, as well as salt, for essential hypertension (Burton 1965:303). Although contemporary medical opinion is divided regarding the dangers of a high sodium diet, doctors at the Hypertension Clinic of New York Hospital agree that such a diet can raise the blood pressure of some people and produce headaches and other symptoms.

13. I agree with Lindenbaum (1977:145) that it would be valuable to repeat this experiment with non-Indian subjects to rule out the possibility that physiological reactions were influenced by anticipations based upon belief in humoral realities.

14. In common with most medical care systems, Malay theory recognizes a multiple series of disease causations of which humoral etiology is only one.

15. This humoral rule provides protection against heat cramps, which can be precipitated by exposure to cold air or water following heavy exercise in the heat (McCullough 1973).

16. According to American doctors I have questioned, salt water aids in surface clotting.

17. Malay fears about the dangers of hospital medicine for measles are based partially on ignorance of the treatment provided. There is no specific medicine for measles; all treatment is symptomatic relying primarily on aspirin for relief of fever and calamine lotion for itch.

18. Malay conceptions regarding measles are similar to those, described by Topley (1976), of Chinese in Hong Kong.

19. These bomoh practice in the best Hippocratic tradition. Although the Hippocratic corpus accepts the concept of the four humors, *On Ancient Medicine* opens: "Whoever having undertaken to speak or write on Medicine have first laid down for themselves some hypothesis to their argument, such as hot, or cold, or moist, or dry, or whatever they choose (thus reducing their subject within a narrow compass, and supposing only one or two original causes of disease or of death among mankind), are all clearly mistaken in much that they say. . . ." (Adams 1886, I:132).

20. For a discussion of the political symbolism of Malay healing, see Kessler (1977).

21. See Dentan (1965) for similar findings among the Semai, an aboriginal people of Malaya.

22. Dietary advice given by bomoh specifically mentioned stale fish rather than stale or impure food in general, in all cases at which I was present.

23. Fresh fish, including bisa species, are neutral with respect to the humoral system.

24. Most of these features have been corroborated by ichthyologists as objectively accurate. Information on feeding habits, however, is problematic. It can be ascertained that many species purported to be bottom feeders actually are as described, but information on other species is lacking. Those described as eating annelid worms and other dangerous organisms are indeed carnivorous (at least those species on which we have information), however, no studies have been done on whether they occasionally eat other organisms besides smaller fish and crustaceans (James Atz 1979, personal communication).

25. Yellow often substitutes for red as symbolic of blood in Malay magic.

26. A number of the criteria for bisa fish are similar to those for "sacred fish" in Hong Kong. They are strong, large fish that are anomalous in appearance and/or behavior (Anderson 1969).

4: CONCEPTION AND PREGNANCY

1. This was noted, as well, by Clive Kessler in Kelantan (Kessler 1979, personal communication).

2. See chap. 6 for the entire jampi in English translation, and Appendix 2 for the original Malay version.

3. For an extensive treatment of these ideas in Acheh, see Siegel 1969.

4. Although hati may be glossed as liver (i.e., *hati ayam* means chicken liver), it is more often used figuratively as the seat of emotions and secret thought, in a manner similar to the English usage of heart.

5. This phrase, *lendir batu*, has a double meaning. It can also be translated as semen of the testicles. See chap. 3 for a discussion of the meanings of lendir. The original Malay version of this incantation is given in Appendix 2.

6. I attempted to have some of these medicines analyzed at the University of Malaya, but was unsuccessful, as a proposal to WHO for funds to support this and allied studies, prepared by the university faculty, was not funded during my stay.

7. This plant is called *ceraka* in standard Malay, from the Sanskrit *chitraka* (Gimlette and Thomson 1971:42; Burkill 1966:1805). Folk etymology in Merchang has endowed the name with meaning previously lacking.

8. Since approximately 15 percent of all pregnancies in the United States end in spontaneous abortion, usually during the early months, and the percentage is probably higher in Third World countries (Potter and

Parker 1964:101), it may well be that abortion would have occurred without the bomoh's intervention.

9. Similar beliefs exist in other Southeast Asian cultures, e.g., Philippines (Cole 1956:69; Ewing 1960:132) and Indonesia (Geertz 1960:46).

10. Eclipses are not feared in Merchang at present. If one occurs, mothers-to-be are advised to tell their unborn children, "Wake up, Missy or Sonny, and look over there" (*Bangun Mek Awang kelih nu*). This keeps the baby from being startled. If she neglects to do so, the child may be somewhat restless, hardly a serious consequence.

11. Dentan (1965) reports similar behavior among the Semai, an aboriginal people of Malaysia.

12. Skeat describes a similar cure using fish bones for lekat kenan caused by a father-to-be who knocked many fish on their heads (1972:349).

13. A variation on this theme can be found in Skeat 1972:432–433.

14. This division into "the raw and the cooked" is a conscious one on the part of Malays. Offering to the spirits of the village and fields include cooked eggs; eggs given to jungle spirits are often raw.

15. Urat is a difficult word to translate since it can mean nerves, blood vessels, or muscles. It is usually impossible to narrow down exactly which is being referred to, as they are thought to be inseparable. Therefore urat may mean one or all these categories, which are separated in English thought.

16. Yellow and red both stand for blood in Malay magic.

5: GOVERNMENT MIDWIFE AND TRADITIONAL MIDWIFE

1. Kuah (1972:84), however, thinks that "most of the practices in relation to pregnancy and childbirth, as practiced by the Malays, do not appear to be medically harmful." He adds that his "is not a true scientific paper inasmuch as the materials are mainly hearsay evidence but in view of the scarcity of reference works on this topic it is felt that the materials collected ought to be recorded in a medical journal."

2. This was true in Chen's study area in Kedah as well, where the median number of postpartum home visits was three (Chen 1975:163).

3. Of all the registered bidan kampung in Malaysia, only three are male (Siti Hasmah 1975a:4).

4. Patients at the General Hospital must also provide their own bottles to be filled at the hospital pharmacy.

5. Health personnel higher up in government echelons recognize that

local health staff frequently have negative attitudes toward traditional birth attendants, and have recommended that they be viewed in a more positive light (Siti Hasmah 1975a:1—2).

6. Although the government midwife does not perform external version, obstetricians in the hospital do. Halimah had her own fetus turned in the hospital late in pregnancy. Since version is performed by Malaysian doctors, the practice in itself cannot be the source of concern. If it is a reasonable procedure when done in the hospital but fraught with danger when performed by a traditional midwife, there must be serious differences in the way it is carried out. I have seen no study detailing these differences, or showing that version done in the hospital is more effective or less hazardous than when performed by bidan kampung. It would be interesting to know how often version done by a traditional midwife results in damage, and to be able to compare these statistics with similar ones from the hospitals.

External version was performed until recently by American obstetricians, who now consider Cesarian section preferable. Opinions vary among American obstetricians as to the possible value of turning the fetus. Some say the fetus will invariably turn back, while others believe version may be effective if done in the eighth month, and is worth trying under circumstances where Cesarian section is unlikely to be performed, because the dangers of version are less than those of breech birth.

7. These procedures will be discussed in chap. 6.

8. When this occurred to the daughter-in-law of a recently deceased bomoh, people ascribed it to her husband's lack of control over his inherited familiar spirits, who kept pushing the baby back into the birth canal.

6: GIVING BIRTH IN A MALAY VILLAGE

1. McHugh gives a jampi for protection against the pontianak collected in Trengganu (1959:80).

2. Dove (*punai*) often refers, in Malay charms, to the patient or his semangat. In this context, however, it refers to the bidan's mixture.

3. The midwife is exhorting the spirits to depart.

4. The original Malay version of this charm is found in Appendix 2.

5. Ancient Egyptians sprinkled salt over the dying and newly dead, hoping to keep the soul within its fleshy envelope. The Jews forbade its use in the chamber of death since they were anxious to free the soul from the body. The practice of rubbing salt on newborn babies, alluded to in

Ezekiel (16:4), was meant to strengthen the new soul's hold on the body and protect the child from evil spirits. Cabalists claim that salt drives away such spirits, and recommend that new homes be inaugurated with bread and salt, a practice still followed by modern Jews. The zombie of Haitian legend is supposed to regain his spiritual autonomy upon ingesting salt. In European witchcraft mythology, salt is conspicuous by its absence from witches' sabbath feasts. The Inquisitor warned his assistants to wear bags filled with salt to protect themselves from their suspects' familiar spirits (Trachtenberg 1977:160—161).

6. Annandale (1903—1904:64) wrote that many bidan in Patani claimed power to bring abnormal births back to their true human form. One wonders how many bidan in those days would have complained that their powers were never allowed to be put to the test, and how many others would have exhibited the tough-minded "show-me" attitude of Sapiah.

7. Actually the direction from Malaysia to Mecca is west northwest. It is recognized by Tok Hitam's table of intrinsic heats as the hottest direction, corresponding to the heat of Friday, the Islamic sabbath.

8. Hantu are frequently referred to as *syaitan* and *iblis* (satan and devil in Arabic) by Malays.

9. Cuisinier (1951:204) writes that the conception of the soul in the form of a bird is the most common belief regarding the soul throughout the Malaysian Archipelago. The Malays' identification of the soul with the chicken (the bird most in evidence in their lives) is shown by the use of the chicken in circumcision feasts, rituals to release a new mother from the postpartum period, and in the frequent representations of chickens at wedding parties. Skeat (1972:587) notes that bomoh of his day called the soul by the sound used to call fowl.

10. This incantation has been incorporated, by the bomoh, into the *Main Puteri*.

11. *Loh mapor*, which I translate as the Book of Fate, is a Malay corruption of the Arabic *luhal mahfudz*, the tablet on which is written all that is to take place up to the Day of Judgment. The Hadith is a collection of traditions about the sayings and deeds of Muhammad.

12. According to medieval Islamic and European theory, as well as present-day Malay thought, the female develops on the left side of the uterus and the male on the right. This theory was expanded by medieval physicians and philosophers to explain occasions on which a fetus which appeared to be located on the right side proved to be female and vice versa: boys developing on the left side were supposed to partake of

feminine traits while girls who developed on the right were suspected of having been masculinized. See Hertz (1960) for further discussion of this question.

13. The concept of sesuai is similar to the Javanese concept of *tjotjog* discussed by Geertz (1960:31).

14. Results of Goland's study are at variance with those of Akil. A different assay technique was employed that showed little change in beta endorphin levels during pregnancy, but significant rises during labor.

15. When this occurred during the birth of a grandchild of a deceased bomoh, the popular diagnosis was that the familiar spirits which the baby's father had inherited were not yet under his control. Their uncontrolled presence allowed them to afflict the vulnerable mother and child.

16. This was the only time I ever observed bamboo used to cut the umbilical cord. All other times a scissors was employed. As the bidan kampung were not in the habit of sterilizing their scissors, a newly cut piece of bamboo might have been the better choice.

17. Although Winstedt writes that for all births "the child is first spat upon by the midwife in order that he may be protected against the old Indonesian spirits of disease" (1951:41), this was the only occasion at which I witnessed such behavior.

7: THE POSTPARTUM PERIOD

1. For analyses of diets, see Appendix 4.

Bibliography

Abdullah bin Abdul Kadir
   1969   *The Hikayat Abdullah.* Translated by A. H. Hill. Kuala Lumpur: Oxford University Press.

Adams, Francis
   1886   *The Genuine Works of Hippocrates.* 2 vols. Translated from the Greek with a Preliminary Discourse and Annotations. New York: William Wood.

Akil, Huda, S. J. Watson, J. D. Barchas, and C. H. Li
   1979   "B-Endorphin Immunoreactivity in Rat and Human Blood: Radioimmunoassay, Comparative Levels and Physiological Alterations." *Life Sciences* 24:1659–1666.

Alland, Alexander, Jr.
   1966   "Medical Anthropology and the Study of Biological and Cultural Adaptations." *American Anthropologist* 68:40–51.
   1970   *Adaptation in Cultural Evolution: An Approach to Medical Anthropology.* New York: Columbia University.

Anderson, Betty Ann, M. E. Camacho, and J. Stark
   1974   *The Childbearing Family.* New York: McGraw-Hill.

Anderson, E. N., Jr.
   1969   "Sacred Fish." *Man* (NS) 4:443–449.
   1980   " 'Heating' and 'Cooling' Foods in Hong Kong and Taiwan." *Social Science Information* 19 (2):237–268.

Annandale, Nelson, and Herbert C. Robinson
   1903–   *Fasciculi Malayenses: Anthropological and Zoological Results of an*
   1904   *Expedition to Perak and the Siamese Malay States 1901–1902.* Liverpool: University Press of Liverpool.

Bibliography

Arms, Suzanne
  1975 *Immaculate Deception: A New Look at Women and Childbirth.* Boston: Houghton Mifflin Co.
Bailey, F. G.
  1969 *Spoils and Strategems: A Social Anthropology of Politics.* New York: Schocken Books.
Barth, Fredrik
  1959 *Political Leadership Among Swat Pathans.* London School of Economics Monographs on Social Anthropology, no. 19. New York: Humanities Press.
Beck, Brenda E. F.
  1969 "Colour and Heat in South Indian Ritual." *Man* (NS)4:553–572.
Birnbaum, David A.
  1978 "Iatrogenesis of Damaged Mothers and Newborns." In *21st Century Obstetrics Now!* Vol. 1. Edited by Lee Stewart and David Stewart. Marble Hill, Mo: NAPSAC Inc.
Bolton, M.
  1972 "Food Taboos among the Orang Asli in West Malaysia." *Am. J. Clin. Nut.* 25:798.
Botha, M.
  1968 "The management of the umbilical cord in labour." *S. Afr. J. Obst.* 6:30–33.
Brown, C. C.
  1935 "Trengganu Malay." *J. Royal Asiatic Soc. Malay Br.* 13 (3): 1–111.
  1951 *Malay Sayings.* Singapore: Asia Pacific Press.
  1970 *Sejarah Melayu "Malay Annals."* Translated by C. C. Brown. Kuala Lumpur: Oxford University Press.
Brown, Roy, R. D. Shaffer, I. L. Hansen, H. B. Hansen, and M. A. Crawford
  1966 "Health Survey of the El Molo." *E. Afr. Med. J.* 43 (11):480–488.
Browne, Edward G.
  1921 *Arabian Medicine.* London: Cambridge University Press.
Burgess, A., and R. Dean
  1962 *Malnutrition and Food Habits.* New York: MacMillan.
Burkill, I. H.
  1966 *A Dictionary of the Economic Products of the Malay Peninsula.* Kuala Lumpur: Ministry of Agriculture and Cooperatives.

Bibliography

Burkill, I. H., and Mhd. Haniff
  1930 "Malay Village Medicine." *The Gardens Bulletin, Straits Settlement*, VI.

Burton, Benjamin T.
  1965 *The Heinz Handbook of Nutrition*. New York: McGraw-Hill.

Cassidy, Claire M.
  1980 "Benign Neglect and Toddler Malnutrition." In *Social and Biological Predictors of Nutritional Status, Physical Growth and Neurological Development*. Edited by Lawrence Greene and F. B. Johnston. New York: Academic Press.
  1981 "Benign Neglect: A Consideration of Some Adaptive Aspects of Toddler Malnutrition." Paper presented at University of Massachusetts (Boston) Symposium on Cultural Aspects of Food and Nutrition.

Chapin, Mac
  1976 "Muu Ikala: Cuna Birth Ceremony." In *Ritual and Symbol in Native Central America*. Edited by Philip Young, and James Howe. University of Oregon Anthropological Papers, no. 9.

Chen, Paul C. Y.
  1972 "Socio-cultural Influences on Vitamin A Deficiency in a Rural Malay Community." *J. Trop. Med. Hyg.* 75:231–236.
  1973 "An Analysis of Customs Related to Childbirth in Rural Malay Culture." *Trop. geog. Med.* 25:197–204.
  1974– "The Malay Traditional Birth Attendant." *Ethnomedizin* 3
  1975 (3/4):335–352.
  1975 "Midwifery Services in a Rural Malay Community." D.M. Thesis, Department of Social and Preventive Medicine, University of Malaya.

Clifford, Sir Hugh
  1898 *Studies in Brown Humanity*. London: Kegan, Ltd.

Cole, Fay-Cooper
  1956 "The Bikidnon of Mindanao." Chicago Natural History Museum Fieldiana, Anthropology, vol. 46.

Colson, Anthony C.
  1971 *The Prevention of Illness in a Malay Village: An Analysis of Concepts and Behavior*. Monograph Series Two. Winston Salem, N.C., Wake Forest University.

Country Report—Malaysia
  1975 Xeroxed copy distributed at International Confederation of

Midwives/International Federation of Gynaecology & Obstetrics, Kuala Lumpur.

Craig, Charles P.
1980 "It's Always the Big Ones That Should Get Away." *J.A.M.A.* 244 (3):272–273.

Cravioto, Joaquin
1958 "Consideraciones Epidemiologicas y Bases Para la Formulacion de un Programa de Prevencion de la Desnutricion." *Bol. Hosp. Inf. Mex.* 15:925–935.

Cuisinier, Jeanne
1936 *Danses Magiques de Kelantan.* Travaux et Memoires de l'Institut d'Ethnologie de l'Université de Paris, 22.
1951 *Sumangat: L'Ame et son Culte en Indochine et en Indonésie.* Paris: Gallimard.

Currier, Richard L.
1966 "The Hot-Cold Syndrome and Symbolic Balance in Mexican and Spanish-American Folk Medicine." *Ethnology* 5:251–263.

Czontos, K., M. Rust, V. Hollt, W. Mahr, W. Kromer, and H. J. Teschemacher
1979 "Elevated Plasma Levels in Pregnant Women and Their Neonates." *Life Sciences* 25:835–844.

Dentan, Robert Knox
1965 "Some Senoi Semai Dietary Restrictions: A Study of Food Behavior in a Malayan Hill Tribe." Ph.D. dissertation, Department of Anthropology, Yale University.

Department of Social and Preventive Medicine, University of Malaya
1968 "Food Composition Tables Compiled for Use in West Malaysia." Unpublished.

De Walt, K. M., P. B. Kelly, and G. H. Pelto
1980 "Nutritional Correlates of Economic Microdifferentiation in a Highland Mexican Community." In *Nutritional Anthropology: Contemporary Approaches to Diet and Culture.* Edited by Norge W. Jerome, Randy F. Kandel, and Gretel H. Pelto. New York: Redgrave Publishing Company.

Djamour, Judith
1966 *The Muslim Matrimonial Court in Singapore.* New York: Humanities Press, Inc.

Douglas, Mary
1966 *Purity and Danger.* London: Routledge and Kegan Paul, Ltd.

Bibliography

Dunn, F. L.
  1975   *Rain-Forest Collectors and Traders: A Study of Resource Utilization in Modern and Ancient Malaya.* Monographs of the Malaysian Branch of the Royal Asiatic Society, no. 5.
Endicott, K. M.
  1970   *An Analysis of Malay Magic.* Oxford: Clarendon Press.
Ewing, Franklin, S.J.
  1960   "Birth Customs of the Tawsug, Compared with Those of Other Philippine Groups." *Anthrop. Quarterly* 33:129–133.
Fabrega, Horacio, Jr.
  1974   *Disease and Social Behavior: An Interdisciplinary Perspective.* Cambridge: MIT Press.
Fabrega, Horacio, Jr., and D. B. Silver
  1973   *Illness and Shamanistic Curing in Zinacantan.* Stanford: Stanford University Press.
Firth, Raymond
  1974   "Faith and Skepticism in Kelantan Village Magic." In *Kelantan: Religion, Society and Politics in a Malay State.* Edited by William R. Roff. Kuala Lumpur: Oxford University Press.
Firth, Rosemary
  1966   *Housekeeping Among Malay Peasants.* New York: Humanities Press (1st ed. 1949).
Foster, George W., and Barbara G. Anderson
  1978   *Medical Anthropology.* New York: John Wiley & Sons.
Frazer, Sir James G.
  1959   *The Golden Bough.* New York: Criterion Books (1st ed. 1890).
Freedman, Maurice
  1954   "A Report on Some Aspects of Food, Health and Society in Indonesia." World Health Organization, unpublished.
Geertz, Clifford
  1960   *The Religion of Java.* New York: Free Press.
Gimlette, John D.
  1971   *Malay Poisons and Charm Cures.* Kuala Lumpur: Oxford University Press (1st ed. 1915).
Gimlette, J. D., and I. H. Burkill
  1930   *The Medical Book of Malayan Medicine.* The Gardens Bulletin, Straits Settlement, VI.
Gimlette, J. D., and H. W. Thomson
  1971   *A Dictionary of Malayan Medicine.* London: Oxford University Press (1st ed. 1939).

Bibliography

Gladwin, Christina H.
1979   "Cognitive Strategies and Adoption Decisions: A Case Study of Nonadoption of an Agronomic Recommendation." *Economic Development and Cultural Change* 28 (1):155–173.

Goland, R. S., S. L. Wardlaw, R. I. Stark, and A. G. Frantz
1981   "Human Plasma B-Endorphin during Pregnancy, Labor, and Delivery." *J. Clin. Endocrin. and Metab.* 52:74–78.

Goodhart, Robert S., and Maurice E. Shils
1973   *Modern Nutrition in Health and Disease.* Philadelphia: Lea & Febiger.

Gordon, Bernard L.
1977   "Fish and Food Poisoning." *Sea Frontiers* 23 (4):218–227.

Gordon, Shirle
n.d.   "Malay Marriage—Divorce in the 11 States of Malaysia and Singapore." *Intisari* II (2):23–32.

Grant, Anne
1977   *Nutritional Assessment—Guidelines for Dieticians.* Seattle: privately printed.

Halimah bt. Mahmud
1975   "Midwifery in Rural Areas—Practice and Problems." Paper delivered at Workshop for the Instruction and Practice of Midwifery (*Benkel Latihan dan Amalan Perbidanan*), Kuala Lumpur.

Halstead, Bruce W.
1959   *Dangerous Marine Animals.* Cambridge, MD: Cornell Maritime Press.
1967   *Poisonous and Venomous Marine Animals of the World.* Washington, D.C.: U.S. Government Printing Office.

Hamid, Wan
1964   "Religion and Culture of the Modern Malay." In *Malaysia.* Edited by Wang Gungwu. Singapore: Donald Moore Books.

Hansen, I. L., R. Brown, R. D. Shaffer, and M. A. Crawford
1966   "Biochemical Findings on the El Molo Tribe." *E. Afr. Med. J.* 43 (11):489–500.

Harris, Marvin
1966   "The Cultural Ecology of India's Sacred Cattle." *Cultural Anthropology* 7:51–59.
1977   *Cannibals and Kings: The Origins of Cultures.* New York: Vintage Books.

Bibliography

Hart, Donn V.
  1969   *Bisayan Filipino and Malayan Humoral Pathologies.* Data Paper,
          no. 76, Cornell University Southeast Asia Program.
Hart, D. V., P. A. Rajadhon, and R. C. Coughlin
  1965   *Southeast Asian Birth Customs: Three Studies in Human Reproduc-
          tion.* New Haven: HRAF Press.
Harwood, Alan
  1971   "Hot-Cold Theory of Disease." *J.A.M.A.* 216 (7):1153–1158.
Hertz, Robert
  1960   *Death and the Right Hand.* Translated by R. and C. Needham.
          New York: The Free Press.
Holmer, Nils M., and S. Henry Wassen
  1953   *The Complete Mu-Igala in Picture Writing: A Native Record of a
          Cuna Indian Medicine Song.* Ethnografiska Musset, Goteborg.
Holvey, David N., and John H. Talbott, eds.
  1972   *The Merck Manual of Diagnosis and Therapy.* 12th edition. Rah-
          way: Merck, Sharp and Dohme Research Laboratories.
Horwitt, M., C. C. Harvey, W. S. Rothwell, J. L. Cutler, and D. Hafron
  1956   "Tryptophan-niacin relationships in man." *J. Nutr.* Supple-
          ment 1:1–43.
Hytten, Frank E., and Isabella Leitch
  1971   *The Physiology of Human Pregnancy.* 2d edition. London: Black-
          well Scientific Publications, Ltd.
Kessler, Clive S.
  1977   "Conflict and Sovereignty in Kelantanese Malay Spirit
          Seances." In *Case Studies in Spirit Possession.* Edited by V. Crap-
          anzano and V. Garrison. New York: Wiley & Sons.
Kleinman, Arthur
  1980   *Patients and Healers in the Context of Culture.* Berkeley, Los
          Angeles, London: University of California Press.
Koran
  1959   Translated by N. J. Dawood. Baltimore: Penguin Books.
Kuah, K. B.
  1972   "Malay customs in relation to childbirth." *Med. J. Malaysia* 27
          (2):81–84.
Laderman, Carol
  1980   "Taming the Wind of Desire." *Asia* 2 (5):34–39.
Lederman, Regina P., E. Lederman, B. A. Work, Jr., and D. S. McCann
  1978   "The Relationship of Maternal Anxiety, Plasma Catechola-

[253]

mines and Plasma Cortisol to Progress in Labor." *Am. J. Obst. Gyn.* 132 (5):495–500.

Lévi-Strauss, Claude
1963*a*   *Structural Anthropology.* New York: Basic Books, Inc.
1963*b*   *Totemism.* Translated by Rodney Needham. Boston: Beacon Press.

Li, Choh Hao
1978   "Chemical Messengers of the Adenohypothysis from Somatotropin to Lipotropin." *Perspectives in Biology and Medicine.* 21:447–464.

Lindenbaum, Shirley
1977   "The 'Last Course': Nutrition and Anthropology in Asia." In *Nutrition and Anthropology in Action.* Edited by Thomas Fitzgerald. Amsterdam: Van Gorcum.
1979   *Kuru Sorcery.* Palo Alto: Mayfield Publishing Co.

Logan, Michael H.
1972   "Humoral Folk Medicine: A Potential Aid in Controlling Pellagra in Mexico." *Ethnomedizin* 1 (3/4):397–410.

McArthur, A. Margaret
1962   *Malaya-12 WHO Assignment Report.* Manila: World Health Organization.

McCullough, John M.
1973   "Human Ecology, Heat Adaptation and Belief Systems: The Hot-Cold Syndrome of Yucatan." *J. Anthro. Research* 29 (1):32–36.

McElroy, Ann, and Patricia K. Townsend
1979   *Medical Anthropology.* North Scituate, Mass.: Duxbury Press.

McHugh, J. N.
1959   *Hantu-hantu: an account of ghost belief in modern Malaya.* Singapore: Eastern Universities, Ltd.

McLean, E. B.
1951   "Iron Therapy in Hypochromic Anemia." *Pediatrics* 7:136.

Mahmud Salim bin Haji Mhd. (Haji)
1975   *Al Iman* (The Faithful). Trengganu Office of Religious Affairs.

Maxwell, Sir George
1907   *In Malay Forests.* Edinburgh: William Blackwood and Sons.

Maxwell, W. E.
1881   "Folklore of Malays." *J. of the Royal Asiatic Soc., Straits Branch* 7:11–29.

Millis, Jean
    1958   "Modifications in Food Selections Observed by Malay Women
            During Pregnancy and After Confinement." *Med. J. Malaya* 13
            (2):139–144.
Montagu, Ashley
    1977   "Social Impacts of Unnecessary Intervention and Unnatural
            Surroundings in Childbirth." In *21st Century Childbirth Now!*
            Vol. 2. Edited by Lee Stewart and David Stewart. Chapel Hill:
            NAPSAC.
Mosely, W. Henry, ed.
    1977   *Nutrition and Human Reproduction*. Washington, D.C.: National
            Institutes of Health.
National Research Council
    1943   *The Problem of Changing Food Habits*. Bulletin 108.
    1974   *Recommended Dietary Allowances*. 8th revised edition. Washing-
            ton, D.C.: National Academy of Sciences.
Newton, Niles
    1977   "Effects of Fear and Disturbances on Labor." In *21st Century
            Obstetrics Now!* Vol. 1. Edited by Lee Stewart and David
            Stewart. Marble Hill, Mo: NAPSAC.
Ngin, C. S.
    1975   "Indigenous Fertility-Regulating Methods in a Chinese Com-
            munity." University of California and International Center for
            Medical Research, Annual Progress Report, San Francisco.
Orso, Ethelyn
    1970   *Hot and Cold in the Folk Medicine of the Island of Chira, Costa Rica*.
            Latin American Studies Division. Baton Rouge: Louisiana
            State University.
Perez, H., C. A. Chavez, and C. Martinez
    1969   "Metodologia Simplificada de Encuestas Nutricionales." *Salud
            Publica de Mexico* 11:223–228.
Perry, Lilly M.
    1980   *Medicinal Plants of East and Southeast Asia: Attributed Properties
            and Uses*. Cambridge: MIT Press.
Peterson, Jean
    1977   "Ecotones and Exchange in Northern Luzon." In *Economic
            Exchange and Social Interaction in Southeast Asia: Perspectives from
            Prehistory, History and Ethnography*. Edited by Karl Hutterer.
            University of Michigan Papers on South and Southeast Asia,
            no. 13.

[255]

Bibliography

Phillips, Herbert P.
  1965   *Thai Peasant Personality: The Patterning of Interpersonal Behavior in the Village of Bang Chan.* Berkeley and Los Angeles: University of California Press.
  1969   "The Scope and Limits of the 'Loose Structure' Concept." In *Loosely Structured Social Systems: Thailand in Comparative Perspective.* Edited by Hans-Dieter Evers. Yale University Southeast Asian Studies. Cultural Report Series, no. 17.

Population and Housing Census of Malaysia
  1970   *Community Groups.* Kuala Lumpur: Jabatan Perangkaan Malaysia.

Potter, Robert G., Jr.
  1963   "Birth Intervals: Structure and Change." *Pop. Studies* 17:155–166.

Potter, R. G., and M. P. Parker
  1964   "Predicting the Time Required to Conceive." *Pop. Studies* 18 (1):99–116.

Provencher, Ronald
  1971   *Two Malay Worlds.* Research Monograph no. 4, Center for South and Southeast Asia Studies, University of California, Berkeley.

Ramanamurthy, P. S. V.
  1969   "Physiological effects of 'Hot' and 'Cold' foods in Human Subjects." *J. Nut. and Diet.* 6:187–191.

Rensberger, Boyce
  1980   "Heat 'Pictures' of Pain Expected to Aid Sufferers, Detect Fakers." *New York Times* 21 October: C3.

Rosina bt. Haji Abdul Karim
  1975   "Historical Review of Midwifery Services and Legislations in Malaysia." Paper presented at Workshop for the Instruction and Practice of Midwifery (*Benkel Latihan dan Amalan Perbidanan*), Kuala Lumpur.

Sahlins, Marshall
  1976   *Culture and Practical Reason.* Chicago: University of Chicago Press.

Sambhi, J. S.
  1968   "Bomoh's Abdomen." *Far East Med. J.* 4:347–348.

Sandosham, A. A.
  1959   *Malariology, with Special Reference to Malaya.* Singapore: University of Malaya Press.

[256]

Bibliography

Schneider, David M.
1968   *American Kinship: A Cultural Account.* Englewood Cliffs, N.J.:
        Prentice-Hall.

Sheppard, M. C.
1949   "A Short History of Trengganu." *J. Royal Asiatic Soc. Malay
        Branch* 22 (3):1–74.

Sherzer, Joel
1974   "Namakke, Sunmakke, Kormakke: Three Types of Cuna
        Speech Event." In *Explorations in the Ethnography of Speaking.*
        Edited by Richard Bauman and Joel Sherzer. London: Cam-
        bridge University Press.

Siegel, James T.
1969   *The Rope of God.* Berkeley and Los Angeles: University of
        California Press.

Siskind, Janet
1973   *To Hunt in the Morning.* New York: Oxford University Press.

Siti Hasmah bt. Mohd. Ali
1968   "The Effect of Islam and Adat on Health Attitudes." Paper
        presented at Malaysian Sociological Research Institute Semi-
        nar, Kelantan.
1975a   "The Role of Traditional Birth Attendants in Family Health."
        Paper presented at Workshop for the Instruction and Practice
        of Midwifery (*Benkel Latihan dan Amalan Perbidanan*), Kuala
        Lumpur.
1975b   "Some Aspects of Traditional Health Attitudes in Rural
        Areas." Paper presented at International Confederation of
        Obstetrics, Kuala Lumpur.

Skeat, W. W.
1972   *Malay Magic: Being an Introduction to the Folklore and Popular
        Religion of the Malay Peninsula.* New York: Benjamin Blom, Inc.
        (1st ed. 1900).

Skeat, W. W., and C. O. Blagden
1906   *Pagan Races of the Malay Peninsula.* London: MacMillan.

Stedman's Medical Dictionary Illustrated
1979   The Williams and Wilkins Co., Baltimore.

Strange, Heather
1971   "The Weavers of Rusila: Working Women in a Malay Village."
        Ph.D. dissertation, Department of Anthropology, New York
        University.

[257]

Tambiah, Stanley J.
1969   "Animals are Good to Think and Good to Prohibit." *Ethnology*
8:423–459.
Teong, T. S.
1975   "Recommended Daily Dietary Intakes for Peninsular Malaysia." *Med. J. Malaysia* 30 (1):38–42.
Thambu, Johan A. M.
1971   "Rupture of the Uterus." *Med. J. Malaysia* 25 (4):293–294.
Thomson, Florence A.
1960   *Child Nutrition—A Survey in the Parit District of Perak*. Bulletin
no. 10, Institute for Medical Research, Kuala Lumpur.
Topley, Marjorie
1976   "Chinese Traditional Etiology and Methods of Cure in Hong
Kong." In *Asian Medical Systems: A Comparative Study*. Edited by
Charles Leslie. Berkeley, Los Angeles, London: University of
California Press.
Trachtenberg, Joshua
1977   *Jewish Magic and Superstition, a Study in Folk Religion*. New York:
Atheneum Press.
Turner, Victor
1964   "Betwixt and Between: the Liminal Period in *Rites de Passage*."
The Proceedings of the American Ethnological Society, Symposium
on New Approaches to the Study of Religion.
U.S. Department of Agriculture
1978   *Food Consumption Prices Expenditures*. Supplement for 1975
Agriculture and Economics Report, no. 138.
Vesey-Fitzgerald, S. G.
1931   *Muhammadan Law, An Abridgement According to its Various
Schools*. London: Oxford University Press.
Whyte, Robert O.
1974   *Rural Nutrition in Monsoon Asia*. London: Oxford University
Press.
Wilkinson, R. J.
1908   *The Incidents of Malay Life*. Part I of Life and Customs, Papers
on Malay Subjects, 1st series. Kuala Lumpur: Government
Printer.
1957   "Malay Customs and Beliefs," *J. Royal Asiatic Soc., Malay
Branch*, 30 (4):1–87.
1959   *A Malay-English Dictionary*. London: MacMillan.

[258]

Bibliography

Wilson, Christine S.

1970 "Food Beliefs and Practices of Malay Fishermen: An Ethnographic Study of Diet on the East Coast of Malaya." Ph.D. dissertation, Department of Nutrition, University of California, Berkeley.

1971 "Food Beliefs Affect Nutritional Status of Malay Fisherfolk." *J. Nutr. Ed.* 2 (3):96−98.

1973 "Food Taboos of Childbirth: The Malay Example." *Ecol. of Food and Nutrition* 2:267−274.

Wilson, C. S., C. White, L. K. Seng, Y. H. Chong, and D. A. McKay

1970 "Relations of Food Attitudes to Nutrient Status in a Malay Fishing Village." *Fed. Proc.* 29:821.

Winstedt, R. O.

1920 "Perak Birth Customs." *J.F.M.S. Museums* 9:84−87.

1951 *The Malay Magician.* London: Routledge & Kegan Paul.

1972a *An Unabridged English-Malay Dictionary.* 4th edition. Kuala Lumpur: Marican & Sons Sdn. Bhd.

1972b *An Unabridged Malay-English Dictionary.* 6th edition. Kuala Lumpur: Marican & Sons Sdn. Bhd.

1972c *The Malays: A Cultural History.* London: Routledge and Kegan Paul (1st ed. 1947).

Wolff, Robert J.

1965 "The Meanings of Food." *Trop. Geog. Med.* 1:45−51.

Wylde, E. Margaret

1956 "Some Superstitious Customs Surrounding Childbirth Noted in Kuala Lumpur." In *Applied Nutrition in Malaya.* Edited by I. A. Simpson. Kuala Lumpur: Institute for Medical Research.

Zainal-Abidin b. Ahmad

1947 "The Various Significations of the Malay word *Sejok*." *J. Royal Asiatic Soc., Malay Branch* 20 (2):41−44.

Index

Abdullah bin Abdul Kadir, 126
Abortifacients, 79−81
Abortion, 45, 78, 79−81, 85, 143−144, 242−243; attitudes of villagers toward, 79, 143−144; and *bomoh*, 81; case study of, 80−81; causes of spontaneous, 82; and Islam, 77, 83; legal status of, 80; medicine to induce, 81; medicine to stop bleeding after, 82; self-induced, 79−80; and traditional midwives, 80
Adaptation: definition of, 1; and dietary conceptions, 21; measures of, 6; of traditional cultures, 3, 4, 101, 102
Afterbirth: burial of, 108, 158, 164; as child's sibling, 85−86, 243; delivery of, 157, 163, 167; as spirit, 98, 129, 201−202
Agta negritoes, 27
Akil, H., 150, 246
Anderson, B. G., 3, 21, 189, 209
Anderson, E. N., Jr., 149, 175, 242
Alland, A., Jr., 3, 4, 102
Angin, 59, 117. *See also* Disease categories, Malay: *Sakit berangin*
Annandale, N., 103, 245

Badi: animals, 96; *badi mayat*, a case study, 97−101; definitions of, 95−96; of human corpses, 96

Bailey, F. G., 2
Barth, F., 2
Belief and behavior, relationship of, 2, 208−209, 211, 212−213; dietary, 3−4, 21−22, 29−32, 212−213
Birnbaum, D. A., 169
Birth intervals: in Merchang, 83; and nursing, 83−84
Birth weights, 196
Bisa, 62−72, 148, 154; and allergy, 64−65; definition of, 62−64; fish, 64, 65, 66−71, 183−184, 186, 228, 230−232, 241, 242; fruits and vegetables, 65, 183−184; speech, 62−63; symbolism of, 64, 67−68, 71−72, 154
Blagden, C. O., 57, 103
Blood tests, 189−196
Bomoh, 9, 18; and care of newborn, 97−98, 100, 174; and childbirth, 140−150, 161, 162, 174; and contraception, 78−79; and humoral treatments, 54, 55−58; and love magic, 19; and pregnancy, 82; prescribes diet, 64, 241; ritual language of, 61−62, 63; specialists, 122−123, 161, 174. *See also* Incantations; *Main Puteri*
Botha, M., 169
Bottlefeeding, 84, 97, 185
Breastfeeding, 12, 97, 185, 188; age at

Index

Divination, 57–58

Divorce, 11, 19; economic consequences of, 17–18; financial obligations of husband after, 16–17; revocation of, 16–17; in Trengganu, 16, 18; woman-instituted, 18

Djamour, J., 105

Douglas, M., 3, 67

Eclipses, 91, 243

Ecology: and diet, 27, 33–34; of Merchang, 9, 10, 23, 27

El Molo, 32

Emotions, denial of, 59–60, 166

Empirical "proofs" of symbolic systems: *bisa*: 68–71, 154; humoral, 37, 41, 47, 49–50, 72, 79–80, 174–175, 240, 241

Endicott, K. M., 60, 212

Ewing, F., 243

Fabrega, H., Jr., 37, 41

Father: 95, 96; behavior during childbirth, 151, 156, 159, 160, 161, 162, 164; behavior during pregnancy, 91–92, 93–94; obligations to children after divorce, 17–18; role in conception, 75–76

Firth, Raymond, 26, 212, 240

Firth, Rosemary, 22, 33, 79

Fish, 21, 22, 209, 228–232. See also *Bisa* fish

Fish poisoning: ciguatera, 69–71; clupiotoxication, 69, 70; scombroid, 65, 69, 70

Flexibility of thought and behavior, 3, 78, 92–93, 171, 182, 186–189, 208–213

Food: avoidances, 63; beliefs and health programs, 31; habits, 1, 3, 11, 30; ideology, 3–4, 21, 22, 29–32; restrictions, compared with taboos, 239. See also Taboos, food

Foster, G., 3, 21, 189, 209

Frazer, Sir J. G., 67

Freedman, M., 187

Fruit, 21, 199; "cold," 46; cultivated, 28–29; "hot," 44, 82; wild, 22–24, 33, 222–223, 239

Geertz, C., 243, 246

Gimlette, J. D., 80, 81, 242

Gladwin, C., 4

Goland, R. S., 150, 246

Goodhart, R. S., 199

Gordon, B. L., 16, 71

Gropper, R., 240

Halstead, B. W., 65, 68, 69, 71

Haniff, M., 81

Hansen, I. L., 32

Harmony: of healer and patient, 98, 148; humoral and *bisa* concepts of, 64, 72; of mother and fetus, 80, 147–148; of person and name, 98–99, 148; of sultan's rule, 60, 61, 62; similarity of Malay and Javanese concepts of, 246

Harris, M., 4

Hart, D., 38, 90

Harwood, A., 37, 41

Health Center (Marang), 8, 91, 97, 100, 112–115, 153

Herbal medicine, 45, 78, 81, 82, 177, 178

Hindu influences, 9–10, 105, 211

Hippocrates, 240, 241

Holvey, D. N., 240

Horwitt, M., 200

Hospital-based medicine, 8, 80, 91, 97, 100, 102, 108, 112, 153, 160, 174, 182, 241, 243, 244; villagers' attitudes towards, 113–144. *See also* Disease categories; Health Center

Humoral beliefs: of Malayan aborigines, 36; and public health programs, 31; in Southeast Asia, 36

Humoral classifications: by age, 38; of food, 44–46, 47, 49, 183; of illnesses, 50–52; of land, water, and metals, 56; of medicines, 38–39, 45, 52–56, 78, 79–81, 82; of seasons, 39; of times of day, 38; by sex, 38; of

Index

treatments, 150, 164–165, 175, 176, 178
Humoral systems: Arabic, 35, 36, 245–246; Chinese, 35, 36, 239; Costa Rican, 37; European, 35–36, 245–246; Indian, 35–36, 37, 50; Latin American, 41; Malay, 35–62; as metaphor, 36, 60–62, 72; Mexican, 37; Puerto Rican, 37, 188
Humors: bodily, 40–41, 68, 174; and childbirth, 150, 153; and diet, 42–48, 183–188; neutral category, 338, 39–40; 47, 181; and newborn, 159; and pregnancy, 41, 74–77, 85; and seasons, 39; and spirit illnesses, 88; and times of day, 38–39, 53–54; and variability, 37–40; and weather, 51
Hytten, F. E., 196, 198

Iddah, 16, 17, 18, 81
Ideology, 1, 3, 92, 172, 208–209, 212, 213. See also Belief and behavior; Bisa; Humoral systems
Incantations, 72, 75, 89, 154, 159, 161; birth, 130, 140–150, 225–226, 227, 244; to change "eggs" into baby, 134; contraceptive, 77–78, 227; postpartum, 206; results of, 149–150
Institute for Medical Research, 44, 49, 190–191
Islam, 9, 13, 15, 36, 62, 95, 142, 144–145; 161, 162, 211, 245; and abortion, 79, 83; and alcohol, 29, 44; attitudes towards traditional midwives, 87, 105; and conception, 85; conflict with Malay folk beliefs, 9–10, 139; food prohibitions of, 27, 28; and marriage, 13–15, 19; ritual purity in, 73–74, 176

Java, 83, 187–188, 246
Jeliffe, D., 208

Kedah, 243
Kelantan, 26, 128
Kelly, P. B., 31

Kenduri, 85, 89, 115, 207, 245
Keras, 88, 99, 160
Kessler, C., 212, 241, 242
Khalwat, 15, 19, 80
Kleinman, A., 5
Kuah, K. B., 184, 243

Labor: behavior of children during, 154, 155, 162; behavior of husband during, 156, 159, 160, 161, 162, 164; expectations of mother's behavior during, 165–166; magical treatments during, 106, 116, 165; physiological and biochemical processes of, 149–150, 246; support from family during, 11, 114, 154–164, 173
Laderman, C., 60, 203
Language: Malay, 9, 210–211; of incantations and rituals, 61–62, 143–147; of royalty, 61–62
Lederman, R. P., 149
Leitch, I., 196, 198
Lenggang perut, 86, 87–90, 105, 115, 118, 129, 160
Lévi-Strauss, C., 71, 145–146
Li, C. H., 150
Lindenbaum, S., 3, 4, 241
Logan, M. H., 37

McArthur, A. M., 93, 105, 123, 184, 185
McCullough, J. M., 37
McElroy, A., 189
McHugh, J. N., 126, 244
McLean, E. B., 169
Madness, 51, 157
Magic, 199, 164–165, 202; childbirth, 159–160, 161, 162, 164–165; love, 19; rice, 25–26. See also Bomoh; Incantations; Language, of incantations and rituals; Main Puteri
Main Puteri, 76, 203, 217
Malay: definition of a, 9; food beliefs and habits compared with American, 29–30; language, 9, 210–211; proverbs, 171, 210, 211
Malayan aborigines: Blandas, 36;

[264]

Index

Semai, 36, 241, 243; Semang, 154
Malaysian Chinese, 8, 9, 79
Malnutrition, 21, 30–31, 208–209;
and ideology, 21, 31, 34, 189–190,
212; and monotony, 22, 31–32;
and poverty, 31, 201. *See also* Diet;
Disease categories, of hospital-
based medicine
Marriage, 12, 20, 176–177; age at
first, 13; *cinabuta*, 17, 80–81;
contract, 15, 18; number of times
married in Merchang, 15; poly-
gynous, 13, 19, 20
Massage: and contraception, 78–79;
during labor, 155, 171; learning to,
115–116; postpartum, 176, 179
Maxwell, Sir G., 123
Maxwell, W. E., 91
May, J., 208
Medical anthropology, 4, 5–7
Menstruation: and intercourse, 74;
and ritual impurity, 73–74; lack of
ritual concerning, 73–74; menarche, 73–74; origin myth, 74; and
pregnancy, 85, 86, 158; Puerto
Rican food prohibitions during,
188; and ritual impurity, 73–74
Merchang: demography of, 26; ecology of, 9, 10, 23, 27; ethnic composition of, 9; housetypes, 10; location, 9
Midwife, government, 9, 86, 112–
113; antenatal care, 109, 113, 120–
122; and contraception, 77; compared with traditional midwife,
167–170; conducting childbirth,
159–164, 166–167; duties of, 106;
home visits of, 106–107, 110; kit of,
161–162; relations with traditional
midwives, 107; relations with villagers, 107, 108–109, 167–169;
training of, 106
Midwife, traditional, 9, 86, 110–120,
122–123, 246; antenatal care, 114,
119–120, 122; attitudes of medical
establishment toward, 104–105,
107, 113, 169, 170–171, 243–244;
compared with government mid-

wife, 167–170; and contraception,
77; kit of, 113, 155; male, 111, 243;
as medical practitioner, 61, 124,
152–165; postpartum recommendations of, 186, 187; regulation of,
105, 112; relations with government midwife, 107–108; reserving
of, 86–87; as ritual specialist, 6,
88–90, 103, 154, 174, 205–207;
supernatural risks to, 117, 205;
training of, 115–119
Millis, J., 37, 64, 184, 185, 186
Monsoon, 16, 22, 179
Montagu, A., 175
Mosely, W. H., 83
Mu-Igala. See Cuna Indians

Newton, N., 149
Nutritional surveys, 30–31, 34

Orso, E., 37

Pahang, 78, 154, 170
Parker, M. P., 83, 243
Patani, 245
Pelto, G. H., 31
Perak, 30–31, 128, 154
Perez, H., 31
Perry, L. M., 80
Peterson, J., 27
Philippines, 90
Phillips, H., 2
Postpartum diet, 186–188; analysis
of, 198–200, 234–247; and ane-
mia, 184–185, 190; fluid restriction
of, 184, 185–186; and thiamine de-
ficiency, 184, 192, 200
Postpartum period, 6; "blues," 98,
202–203; food restrictions, 66,
179, 183–188, 212; hemorrhage,
112–113, 114, 121, 187; psychosis,
98, 203; release from, 115, 118,
182, 204–207
Potter, R. G., Jr., 83, 243
Pregnancy: ages of women at first, 14;
diet during, 29, 82, 90; external
version, 113, 114, 244; fetal devel-

opment, 86; food cravings, 75, 90–91; illegitimate, 80–81; male, 75–76; and medicine, 45; molar, 133; prenatal influences, 90–102; signs of, 85; striations of, 128, 129. See also *Lenggang perut*
Prenatal influences. See Pregnancy
Provencher, R., 64

Rajadhon, P. A., 90
Ramanamurthy, P. S. V., 50
Recommended Dietary Allowances, 197–199
Release, ritual of, 87, 89, 115, 182, 202, 204–207
Rensberger, B., 240
Rice: as food, 21, 22, 32, 48, 209; growing magic for, 25–26; ritual use of, 57, 58, 87–88, 89, 129, 130–131, 159, 162, 163, 205–206
"Roasting bed," 159, 176, 179–182; number of hours used daily, 179–180; removal of, 205–207; use in other Southeast Asian groups, 36
Robinson, H. C., 103
"Rules to break rules," 3, 101, 208, 212, 213

Sahlins, M., 4
Salt: as criterion for humoral "heat," 43, 45, 53–54; and hypertension, 241; ritual use of, 133, 154, 158, 159, 244–245
Sambhi, J. S., 104, 170
Sandosham, A. A., 56
Sayang. See Harmony
Schneider, D. M., 3
Semangat, 244; calling, 140; danger of weakened, 96, 126, 127, 144, 201; equivalence of human and non-human, 89; *nasi semangat,* 89; pervasiveness of, 89, 144; *semangat padi,* 26; strengthening baby's, 99, 157; strengthening mother's, 89, 129, 203
Sesuai. See Harmony
Seven Celestial Midwives, 132
Sexual intercourse: importance of

tight vagina, 176–177; during menses, 74; oral, 151; during pregnancy, 157; during postpartum period, 204; symbolic, 126–128
Sheppard, M. C., 8
Shils, M. E., 199
Siegel, J. T., 11, 242
Silver, D. B., 37
Siskind, J., 3
Siti Hasmah, 37, 104, 105, 112, 170, 182, 184, 185, 243, 244
Skeat, W. W., 25, 57, 63, 91, 95, 103, 126, 135, 176, 179, 183, 243, 245
Smith, C. L., 68, 69
Spirits, 52, 159, 163, 164, 174, 244, 245, 246; afterbirth as, 98, 129, 201–202; *bajang,* 128; *bidandari,* 132; and childbirth, 26, 130–131, 159, 163–164; and disease, 10, 60, 61; earth spirits, 74, 103, 125–126, 130, 201; *Hantu Meroyan,* 201–202, 203–204; *Hantu Raya,* 60, 125; and humors, 56–58; *langsuir,* 126, 127–128; nature of, 125; origin of, 124; *pelesit,* 111; *penanggalan,* 126–127, 129–130; *pontianak,* 126, 127–128; and postpartum period, 201–204, 206; and pregnancy, 87–88, 89, 96
Startle reaction, 94, 127, 157
Stone, B. C., 224
Strange, H., 105
Sultan, 60, 62, 88, 90–91, 131; as cooling influence, 61, 62, 72; language of, 61–62, 63
Swettenham, F., 210
Symbolism, 3, 4, 72, 78, 88, 148–149, 208, 212, 213; of *bisa* concept, 64, 67–68, 61, 72, 154; in childbirth, 148–149, 151, 162–163; of herbal medicine, 178; of humoral systems, 36, 60–62, 72. *See also* Conception; Incantations; *Keras; Lenggang perut;* Magic

Taboos, food, 21, 27, 63, 92, 184, 189; compared with *pantang* and food restrictions, 63, 239; explained by

Designer: UC Press Staff
Compositor: Trend Western
Printer: Thomson-Shore
Binder: John H. Dekker and Sons
Text: Baskerville
Display: Bodoni